NAVIGATING THE PRESCHOOL YEARS

Sleep, Behavior & Development for 3 to 6 Year Olds

Little Ones

littleONES

The information contained in this book is intended to be used as a guide only and is not intended to replace an individualized consultation by a qualified health professional. If you have any concerns about your child's health or behavior, please consult with your qualified health professional.

ISBN: 978-0-473-64656-1

To Charlie and Kenzie; the little ones.

Where would we be without you.

CONTENTS PAGE

ABOUT THIS BOOK

In late 2015 two mothers, who were also friends, started talking about the idea of a company where parents can access reliable, trusted, proven advice and methods to help their children sleep better, without having to spend a fortune on private consultants, without limiting the support a person can get to the area they live in.

The idea for Little Ones was born.

These mothers knew what sleep deprivation was like. They knew how it felt to struggle through endless sleepless months, wondering what was going on, questioning and doubting themselves at every turn. They knew how long those nights were and how the tears flowed easily during the day too. They'd had babies who were bad night sleepers, bad daytime nappers, babies who were rocked to sleep, fed to sleep, bounced to sleep. Babies who slept in the stroller, front pack, hammock, their arms. Babies who were breast and bottle fed, babies who woke at 5 AM every single day. They'd had days where they couldn't see through the fog. Where everything was just a bit too hard. A lot too hard, if they're being honest.

Everything was a battle; motherhood, their relationships with their husbands, their day to day lives. And it was a battle because they had no idea what to do! They had no idea what was coming next - they were on the back foot 100% of the time. Looking back now, they can see straight away how their lives could have been so different. How their first taste of motherhood could have been so much more enjoyable if they'd had the knowledge, the education about settling and sleep, reliable advice and age-appropriate methods...

And this is why they started their company - to help people. To help people see through that fog, to give families an alternative to sleep deprivation, to let everyone know that there is another way and with the right advice and a village behind you - anything is possible.

Amanda and Nicky, now Pediatric Sleep Experts and having helped over 200,000 families worldwide through their hugely successful Little Ones App, have joined forces with trained child psychologists to bring you this detailed book, specifically written to guide you through the challenging ages of 3 to 6 years. In it you'll find scientifically backed information on the world of child sleep, strategies to help with bedtime settling, night sleep and waking, bedwetting and more. There is information on dealing with tantrums and big changes in your child's life. You are walked through your child's developmental stages and taught how to best help your little one in this rapid period of growth and change.

But that's not all! Inside the Little Ones App we have programs, schedules, trackers, methods, troubleshooting, advice and live sleep consultants for babies from birth to 3 years old, so if you have a baby or toddler at home, or know someone who does, head to our website and enjoy a 10% discount by using the code LITTLEONES4SLEEP - www.littleones.co

SECTION 1:

Sleep

THE IMPORTANCE OF SLEEP

At this time in your little one's life, they are growing and developing at an extremely rapid rate. Sleep is more important now than it's ever been, to assist in all this physical, mental and emotional development.

But, as we all know, sleep can come with its own unique set of challenges between the ages of 3 and 6.

In this book, we delve into the sometimes complex world of sleep for your little person. A world of sleep that is now becoming linked to behavior, habit, ritual and negotiation. We will also explore the other elements coming into play for them in this big period of change - tantrums, emotions, boundaries, and how we can help our children grow into emotionally capable, confident humans.

Let's start by discussing how much sleep your child ought to be having.

By the age of around 3, your little one has ideally dropped their daytime nap altogether (for more info on this, see the section "What to Do When Naps Run Out"). This means you're left with all your sleep eggs in the overnight basket. To aim for great night sleep, don't be afraid of an early bedtime! Many children in this age bracket are being put to bed quite late and this in itself can be a leading cause of poor sleep and troubling behavior during the day.

This is what your little one's sleep should look like:

3 years old	Bedtime 6:30-7:00 PM
4 years old	Bedtime 7:00 PM
5 years old	Bedtime 7:00 PM
6 years old	Bedtime 7:00-7:30 PM

If your child is having significantly less sleep than this, they might be experiencing some or all of the following:

- Lots of tantrums or meltdowns during the day
- Argumentative behavior
- Lack of interest in food
- Wanting/trying to fall asleep in the afternoon or early evening
- Severe irrationality
- Difficulty settling at bedtime
- Lack of focus or concentration during the day

You see, sleep lays the foundation from which every part of our daily lives stems. Often, a lot of the "negative" behaviors our children display comes from overtiredness and in some cases, chronic sleep deprivation.

In this book you will learn how to help your little one achieve the sleep they need for a healthy body and mind in a calm, respectful manner.

SLEEP HORMONES

To start exploring the world of sleep, you firstly need to understand how sleep works. Sleep is a very natural process that is governed biologically by the production and release of a couple of crucial hormones - melatonin and cortisol - and it can just as easily be sabotaged by these hormones too!

Let's take a look at how these hormones help your child to sleep...

Melatonin

As a child nears bedtime in the evening, they start to experience a rise in melatonin levels. Melatonin is often referred to as "the sleep hormone". It is released in the dark and is responsible for us falling asleep and staying asleep.

Melatonin governs our night-time sleep cycles (which are longer than daytime sleep cycles) and differentiates night sleep from day sleep in our brains. Traditionally speaking (before we were able to prolong daylight via electric lights) as dusk approached and the daylight diminished, our bodies would have started to release this hormone, making us sleepy leading up to bedtime. Melatonin is only released in the dark. This is why the natural, biological bedtime for babies and children tends to be between 6:30 PM to 7:30 PM – just after dusk.

During summer months when the sun sets a lot later, many babies and young children struggle to settle and sleep if their room is still too sunny and bright. This is because the sleep hormones are not being released to tell them it is time for night-time sleep; they can't switch into their night-time sleep cycles. We can get around this by creating a false night with blackout blinds or dark curtains.

Once asleep, the melatonin continues to rise in our bodies until around midnight. This is why the period between bedtime and midnight is considered the most restorative sleep - we are being pumped full of those good sleep hormones. After midnight the melatonin drops off, which can mean many children sleep well up until midnight then wake every 2 hours beyond that (especially if they can't self-settle or if something is bothering them).

By around 5:00 AM the melatonin has pretty much gone out of our systems. This is the end of our night-time sleep cycles, and we enter a period of light sleep rather than the deep sleep we were in previously. Here, if anything is bothering your child such as thirst, getting a bit cold, hearing noises or they are unwell, they will really struggle to go back to sleep.

Cortisol (affectionately known as "The Stress Hormone")

Cortisol is a hormone that builds up during our waking hours and is a very natural part of our daytime cycle. Cortisol levels naturally increase in the day and are then reduced when we nap, relax or overnight. In large doses, cortisol is similar to adrenaline or caffeine in the way it affects our bodies, so we don't want the levels to get too high in our children because it will really affect their sleep. High levels of cortisol can inhibit the release of melatonin, meaning your child won't be getting the good sleep hormones they need to go into a deep sleep overnight.

Overtiredness is a key cause of elevated cortisol and this might be happening if your little one is sleeping poorly at night or waking really early in the morning. Napping during the day is one way to reduce the levels of cortisol, as is having some quiet relaxation time for children who no longer nap. It is important our little ones have this downtime because high levels of cortisol will cause hyperactivity (common overtired behavior) and will make it very hard for our children to switch off and go to sleep. It would be like having a cup of coffee right before bedtime and then trying to sleep.

Another cause of elevated cortisol is stress. Now, in your child, this might be different to how you see stress yourself. Your little one might genuinely get stressed if they don't have their favorite cup at lunchtime or if they are not allowed to watch TV any longer. Any situation or behavior that causes your child to cry or have a tantrum is likely increasing their cortisol levels. Now, we're not saying to just give your child what they want all the time to avoid any kind of stress! Let's be honest, children this age stress themselves out easily enough. But being mindful of when your child is stressed is important. If a tantrum occurs right before bedtime in the evening, you will be pretty unsuccessful getting your little one to go to sleep due to the elevated cortisol. Being mindful of this is more about doing what it takes to avoid stress or meltdowns from your little one at key moments, like right before bed. For more information on how to handle this behavior, read the tantrums section further on in this book.

OVERTIREDNESS

When your child is overtired, their system sort of goes into overload and they need to have a sleep so their overactive brain has a chance to process and catch up. This is how they grow and learn.

If your child is overtired, this is what it looks like:

1. crying frequently over any little thing and difficult to calm down
2. they seem hyperactive or like they have a second wind
3. tantrums
4. refusing to eat
5. finding it difficult to fall asleep at bedtime at night
6. waking a lot in the night
7. waking early morning

What is actually happening in your child's body is a buildup of the hormone cortisol. An overload of this is similar to adrenaline and works like caffeine in your little one's system. This is why children can seem suddenly so wide awake - it's like they've just had a shot of coffee right before bedtime. Cortisol inhibits the production and release of another hormone - melatonin - which is the one we actually need in order to settle well and stay asleep. The more overtired your child is, the less likely they are to then settle easily. If they're overtired at bedtime in the evening, they're starting off the night on the back foot and you're pretty much guaranteed a bedtime battle, a bad night of restless sleep then an early wake the next morning.

Many things can cause your child to be become overtired:

- late nights
- nightmares or wakeful sleep
- sleep apnoea
- waking too early in the morning
- having extremely active days with little down time and a bedtime that is a bit too late

It becomes quite obvious when our little ones are overtired - they will be grouchy, unreasonable, argumentative, then the next minute they'll have boundless energy. The only real cure for overtiredness (other than avoiding it in the first place) is sleep. Early bedtimes are more advantageous than offering naps in this age group because a nap can then really wreak havoc on your child's sleep that night, in turn causing more overtiredness!

Don't be scared of an early bedtime.

Contrary to popular belief, an early bedtime won't necessarily correlate to an earlier wake up time the next morning... but a late bedtime (and an overtired child) will likely cause an earlier start the next day.

WHAT TO DO WHEN THE NAPS RUN OUT

Somewhere around the age of 3, your little one will stop napping altogether. This is a dark day! If your child is over 3 and is still having a nap during the day, this can be fine unless it's starting to interfere with their night time settling and sleep. Signs that your little one needs their nap cut down in length, then removed altogether are:

- Taking a long time to settle to bed in the evening and/or bedtime is having to be quite late (later than 8 PM)
- Waking multiple times overnight and/or staying awake for long period in the night
- Waking very early in the morning

If any or all of these things are happening for your child, we would recommend first ensuring their nap is starting no later than 12:30 PM, then cutting their nap in length every few days until it's half an hour long, then removing it altogether.

As the nap is vanishing, we do still suggest offering it perhaps every second day, then maybe twice a week while your little one gets used to the new routine.

Definitely bring bedtime in the evening earlier to compensate and don't be scared of a 6:30 PM bedtime!

Once the nap is gone altogether, you will need to replace "nap time" with "quiet time". Your little one will still require some down time during their busy day. Our recommendation is to keep this at the same time the nap used to happen, so say 12:30-1:30 PM, and ideally in your child's room.

Quiet time activities might include:

- Reading
- Drawing
- Listening to an audio book
- Listening to music
- Building blocks
- Mindfulness/meditation

Think of activities that are "quiet" in their nature, relaxing and don't require physical or mental exertion. This quiet time is a nice chance for your little one to catch up and have a breather.

As your child gets older, quiet time can be done independently. Once you've helped them learn the building blocks of what quiet time entails, they are well capable of spending that time independently in their room, pottering away at their quiet time activities.

This is great for 2 reasons. Firstly it helps encourage independence in your little one. It is important that our children learn to be comfortable with their own company as it builds their self-confidence and independent life skills. Secondly, if your little one is managing their own quiet time, you are able to have a bit of a break yourself - this is crucial to your own wellbeing when you're a parent of a busy child.

Quiet time works best when it's role modeled. If you have a younger baby or toddler in the house, they'll ideally still be napping during the middle of the day, so that's their quiet time. Your 3-6 year old child is having their quiet time, and we recommend you also use this time to engage in a peaceful, mindful activity of your own.

BEDTIME

Once your little one is no longer napping in the day, they can and will need an early night! Being a pre-schooler is exhausting, especially if you're also at daycare or school. Couple that with the massive growth that happens across this period, throw in some big life changes such as a new sibling or starting a new school and it's a recipe for a very tired little person.

Don't be scared of an early bedtime. An appropriate bedtime to aim for between the ages of 3-6 years old is 7 PM.

That said, if your child has had a big day, an early start or just generally seems overly tired, it's totally fine to put them to bed anytime between 6-7 PM. Contrary to what might seem logical, an earlier bedtime doesn't necessarily mean an earlier wake up time in the morning, in fact, a late bedtime and/or an overtired child is the main contributing factor to early rising.

Let's look at some key elements to ensure your little one is heading towards a nice and easy early bedtime of around 7 PM, including ideas for a good bedtime routine:

1. No Screens!

In the 2 hours up until bedtime, try and avoid screen time for your child - this means TV as well as phone or tablet screens. The reason for this is that you're endeavoring to wind your child's brain down, and blue/white light, flashing animated images and stimulating sounds are doing the exact opposite! It will be a lot harder for your child to wind-down to sleep if they're exposed to screens within the 2 hours before bed.

2. Unwind Time

Instead of TV or a game on your phone, have a nice relaxing wind-down routine prior to bed. Doing this in the period between dinner and bedtime is the ideal time. Some good wind-down activities include reading, listening to relaxing music, mindfulness or meditation, talking together or telling stories, singing, playing quiet games such as puzzles or building blocks, and of course lots of snuggles.

This wind-down time is also a great opportunity for some one-on-one interaction, to squeeze in lots of quality time with your little one before bed. This is especially important if you've been working away from home during the day. Having this concentrated period of one-on-one time in the evening means you're "filling your child's tank" of affection and interaction, meaning they're less likely to request you multiple times after being put to bed or overnight. It helps mitigate any separation anxiety that can occur at bedtime.

3. No Sugar

Just as you wouldn't have a shot of coffee or an energy drink right before bed, definitely don't give your child a sugary snack or drink prior to bedtime. Processed sugar is a massive stimulant for children, especially young children, and can really inhibit the success of them going to bed at a decent hour and then also the quality of their sleep.

A great bedtime snack (if your child has to have one) is a banana. Bananas contain an enzyme called tryptophan which actually helps your little one sleep!

Some other pre-bed snack ideas are:

- Toast (plain or with peanut butter)
- Milk
- Porridge
- Cheese and crackers

4. Calming Sleep Environment

The room in which your child sleeps can often make or break the success of bedtime in your household. Think about what you yourself like in a sleep sanctuary and realize your child is no different. Perhaps you like a very dark room, a particular temperature, nothing noisy or stimulating. Try and recreate this for your little one. Some tips for a really sleep inducing sleep sanctuary are:

- A nice dark room and use of a nightlight only if necessary (ie if your child has expressed a fear of the dark)
- No noisy toys or flashing mobiles that might stimulate your child right when they're trying to get in the zone for sleep
- A comfortable mattress and age-appropriate bedding. This might mean that your 3 year old remains in a toddler sleep sack until they're confident pulling up the blankets themselves.
- An appropriate temperature for sleep - we'd recommend around 20 degrees celsius (68 degrees fahrenheit)
- Think about using white noise if your little one struggles to switch off, has an active imagination or if there are other sounds in your household (ie older siblings or a new baby) that might distract your child from the important task of falling asleep.

BEDTIME BATTLES

Sometimes, for whatever reason, no matter how "perfect" your lead-up is, bedtime can suck. The older our children get, the more clued up they become to the fact that they can, to an extent, control the situations they're in. Bedtime is a classic example. Your little one may no longer view bedtime as an inevitable situation where you are in charge and they come to view bedtime as a game, as a way to exert their own control over what is happening. This will be evident in the ten million questions you get asked at bedtime only, or the four thousand times your littlie gets up right after you put them to bed to ask for water or a snack or one more story. They've realized they can manipulate the system!

Here, it is vitally important for them to start learning boundaries and expectations. Have a conversation with them (during the day) about your bedtime expectations and roleplay the response you require of them at bedtime. Help them play "bedtime" with their toys, where they put their toys to bed in a gentle, calm manner and discuss this in relation to your expectations of your child.

Decide, as a family, what your level of tolerance is around bedtime shenanigans. Will you tolerate a couple get-ups per night? Will you insist your child stays in their room, full stop, as soon as you put them to bed? And then, whatever your goal, work some strategies into it.

Let's explore some options here for bedtime strategies, then we'll look at which strategies might suit the most common bedtime antics:

Check Method

If you're confident your child is good and ready for bed at bedtime (ie they are not overtired) and they are fluffing around or have gotten into the habit of having you in the room with them while they go to sleep, you can use this method.

What you do is proceed as per normal for their bedtime routine, reading a story or singing a song. Stay in the room with them but once they're in bed, give an excuse to leave – reassuring them you're coming back. For example:

"I just have to make a cup of tea, I'll be right back"

Leave the room for 1 minute then come back and praise them for waiting. Then give another excuse to leave, such as:

"Oh, I forgot to put the milk in my tea. I'll be right back."

Leave for 2 minutes then come back.

Continue doing this and each time stay out of the room for longer. Always come back because you're reinforcing the trust that you'll come back to them. The hope is that they'll fall asleep while you're out of the room, because you'll be extending the periods you're out by 1 minute each time.

The next morning it is important to tell them:

"I came back last night and you'd fallen asleep! That's ok – I was so proud of you for going to sleep on your own".

You will need to do this for a few nights before your child is comfortable simply falling asleep once you've left the room the first time.

If your child is getting out of bed and coming to see you, rather than demanding your presence in their room, you can say:

"I will come back and check on you in 5 minutes"

This should keep them in bed, waiting for you to come back. Eventually they'll fall asleep.

A simpler version of this method is to put your little one to bed and say you'll come back in 2/3/5/10 minutes to check on them. The first couple nights, come back while they're still awake so they know you did it - just give them another kiss goodnight and say you'll come back in XX minutes again. But don't. In the morning tell them:

""I came back last night and you'd fallen asleep!"

After a couple nights, don't go in for the first check. If they call out or ask if you're coming, say something like:

"Yep, in 2 more minutes".

Because your little one has virtually no concept of concrete time yet, they'll accept this response and will be asleep in no time. In the morning reiterate that you came in and they'd gone to sleep!

This method can work for a child even right up until 7 or 8 years old.

Silent Returns

If your child, who is normally capable of going to sleep fine, is getting out of bed once you've put them to bed, you can do what is called a "silent return".

You'd implement this method as soon as they got out of bed.

To do a silent return you simply return your child to their bed without any communication. If they talk to you, ignore them. Say nothing. Take them back to their bed and lay them down again.

This can take a few attempts (realistically a thousand). What you are teaching your little one is that their behavior is not being rewarded by a response from you. Even a negative response is still a response and will reinforce the behavior.

You're making their effort not worth the while; you're making it boring for them to get up. And so eventually they'll stop doing it.

You can couple this method with the Check Method, whereby you'd do a silent return then tell them you'll come to check on them in 2/5/10 minutes.

COMMON BEDTIME BATTLES & SOLUTIONS

Fear of the dark

Somewhere around 2-3 years old, imagination fully develops and can take hold quite majorly! You might notice your little one engaging in more imaginative play or roleplay and, while this is awesome, imagination can have its challenges too... Cue fear of the dark. Now, being afraid of the dark isn't something we're born with, in fact mammals innately like the dark as it's comforting and safe, but, when you combine an overactive imagination, the urban legends from older siblings, a couple spooky moments on a favorite TV show or some playground dialogue at pre-school, your child can quite quickly develop a real, aggressive fear of the dark.

The easiest way to tackle this is with the introduction of a night light and/or a special new toy or cuddly to "look after" your little one during the night. Many children prefer to sleep with their bedroom door ajar or open at this age and that's also something you might want to consider.

Making "monster spray" is another option - you can easily do this using hairspray or deodorant spray and spraying it in the room before bed (with your little one looking on) to get rid of anything scary.

Needing Things

Bedtime can bring with it a sudden overwhelming thirst or starvation for our children.... (I know you're rolling your eyes along with me!). The way our children desperately need one more drink or 10 more stories or "my favorite toy" (that one they haven't played with in months) at bedtime never ceases to amaze me. It's all just delay tactics. If you've got a child who insists they need things at bedtime here are some strategies for that:

- Make a checklist of the common "things" and tick it off *before* bed (include water, snack, favorite toy, one more kiss for daddy/the cat/the sofa etc)
- Use the check-in method to stretch out your response time to their demands

Not staying in their room

Getting out of bed the second they're put in it is a really common and very frustrating thing our little ones do! If your child is getting up once they've been put to bed at night (and before they've gone to sleep), we advise the following methods:

- Check-in method
- Silent returns
- Sticker/reward chart for staying in bed

Room/Bed aversion

This scenario is a bit more serious and can require a longer process to remedy. A room or bed aversion can happen when your little one gets a big fright or has a negative experience with either their bedroom or their bed and associates their room/bed with being afraid.

In my own children this has happened when my eldest was 3 and the cat was trapped in her room at bedtime (without us knowing) and she got really afraid. In my youngest, she started having nightmares following a stint in hospital (understandable) and started to associate the nightmares with her bed and her room.

In both cases, my girls began to scream at bedtime, absolutely resisted staying in their beds, waking many many times at night and wanting me or my husband to stay in their room with them. They had very obvious fear.

In these extreme cases, the first thing you have to do is remove the fear altogether and remove the fear from being associated with sleep. This meant, for both girls, removing them from their own bedrooms, as that's what they'd associated the fear with.

Once they realized they didn't have to sleep in their own room, the relief in them was so obvious.

For us, and the advice we'd give you here in this situation too, is that it is a relatively long process, but well worth putting in the time and effort. It looks like this:

a. Remove your child from the source of their fear, ie their bed or their room. If possible put them in with a sibling or even in your own room. The main thing is to remove the fear so they can at least start to sleep again and stop associating fear with sleep.

b. Once they're back into a "normal" sleep pattern (and this might take a few months even), broach the subject of moving back into their own room; make it a positive experience and you definitely need to wait until they're ready. Don't rush it.

c. Let them choose some things for their room to help them reacclimate - a special new cuddly toy, a nightlight, some new blankets. If you can, rearrange their furniture so the room looks and feels a bit different.

d. Move them back into their own room. In an extreme situation, camping in their room with them while they adjust is a possibility. Or, have an older sibling sleep in the room with them for a while.

e. Use lots of positive reinforcement and do not get mad or angry with them if they regress! Even though we might think their fear is ridiculous, it's a big and very real deal to them so we need to respect those feelings.

f. You might have to sit with them while they fall asleep or use the check-in method at bedtime for a little while and/or overnight during the readjustment period.

NIGHT SLEEP CHALLENGES

Children are smart and they understand far more than we give them credit for. They are also creatures of habit and are very strongly governed by their desires, especially prior to 6 or 7 years old. You will know by now that your little one has a different interpretation of the world than you do; theirs is largely grounded in instinct and routine.

Your child understands steps in a process. It is the one thing they are extremely skilled at – cause and effect. They very quickly learn a set of behaviors around sleep that makes it infuriating for the poor person trying to settle them.

Babies, toddlers and children are products of their learning. It is up to us to make sure we are teaching them the behaviors we want them to exhibit, through all our interactions with them.

This section of the Program talks you through your options when it comes to tackling a behavioral settling issue or a night waking habit with your child.

Behavioral or Habit Wakes

Children wake at night for many reasons - they are too hot, too cold, they are sick, they are tangled in their blankets, they've had a bad dream, they need to pee... These are what we'd call "normal" wakes and are to be expected in your little one. In most of these cases, you'll just have to address the issue and pop your child back to bed.

However, waking can occur in children between the ages of 3-6 caused by other factors that need a bit of work, such as your child can't go to sleep without your help, and/or your child has a habit wake.

If your child is relying on you to actively settle them back to sleep by rocking or patting, or by your presence in the room when they go to sleep, you will need to teach them to settle using one of the methods in the "Independent Sleep" section.

In regards to habit waking, ie, your child has the ability to fall asleep unassisted but wakes around the same time every night and calls out to or comes into you, the best way to deal with this is by the silent return method explained in the Bedtime Battles section, where you take your child back to their bed in silence.

There are three main factors that trigger a habit waking response in us all: sunlight, food and communication. If your child is used to getting food or some form of communication in the night it stimulates a body clock trigger, like an alarm clock, which will continue to go off night after night. The best way to deal with this is to refuse them the stimuli in the first place.

For a habit wake using the silent return method, you'll need to persevere with the method for a good few nights. You're teaching your little one that their waking isn't being rewarded with a response from you.

A sticker reward chart is also an excellent way to encourage your little one to stay in their bed. This can be explained in the daytime and reinforced in a positive way each morning. If your child is getting no response from you for their waking in the night yet is receiving a great response from you in the morning for not waking, they will definitely choose the behavior that elicits the better response!

We have some sticker charts available on our website you

can download and print out for your little one by visiting here: www.littleones.co/3to6years

INDEPENDENT SLEEP METHOD

If your child isn't falling asleep on their own and is relying on help from you in some way ie. your presence in the form of cuddling, stroking or laying with them while they fall asleep you can use this method to help them start to fall asleep more independently.

Your presence can be a very strong sleep association, so this transition needs to be treated delicately. We have to be careful not to give your child mixed messages.

This method is made up of several phases which you will follow in this order:

1. Sitting on a chair next to your child's bed while they try to go to sleep. If they get upset, you'll use touch and your voice to soothe them.
2. Move your chair halfway across the room, still using your voice to soothe.
3. Move your chair to the door, still using your voice to soothe.
4. Leave the room, if your child becomes upset use voice to soothe, then leave the room again.

The times indicated for this method are approximate only – some children do it a lot quicker. You should move onto the next phase when your child is ready, rather than focusing too heavily on the days specified in the method but make sure you are progressing through the stages.

Below is a table of the phases and following is a breakdown of the step-by-step instructions for each stage.

Stage One	Touch/Voice to soothe next to child's bed at bedtime	Cuddle to sleep overnight
Stage Two	Voice to soothe at bedtime from halfway across the room	Cuddle to sleep overnight
Stage Three	Voice to soothe at bedtime from the doorway	Cuddle to sleep overnight
Stage Four	Voice to soothe at bedtime from outside the door (if needed)	Voice to soothe overnight

Stage One

<u>Touch to soothe at bedtime, next to your child</u>

1. Start pre-bed wind down routine 15 minutes before bedtime.
2. Take your child to their room, close the curtains.
3. Put your child in their sleeping bag and/or place them in their bed.
4. Implement a sleep phrase here, such as *"It's sleep time now"*.
5. Place a chair in the room and sit right next to your child's bed. Reassure them with the sleep phrase once you're sitting there. If the room is dark, they won't be able to see you very well, but they will still smell, hear and sense your presence.
6. Allow them to try and settle herself to sleep without any

interruption from you. It is important you give them the chance to try and do this on their own. If they start becoming upset*, set a timer for 6 minutes (or a time you're comfortable with).

7. If your child needs help to calm down, you can use your voice or touch to help soothe your child, for the duration of the timer. Once calm, stop your timer and again allow your child to try and settle herself without interruption. Repeat the process if they start to become upset until your child has fallen asleep. If your child is still upset after the timer is up you can use touch to soothe them until calm.
8. If your child is awake but happy, leave them to it - no need to repeat the sleep phrase, just stay beside them until they fall asleep. The message you are sending your child is that you are still there to soothe them while they learn to go to sleep on their own, in their own bed.
9. Once your child has fallen asleep in their own bed, no matter how long it takes, that is a massive first step!
10. The first day and night are the hardest as you both adjust to the new way of doing things.
11. Overnight, put your child back to sleep using whatever method you used previously (patting, cuddling) for the time being.

The most important thing at this point is that your child is learning to go to sleep, on their own, in their own bed at the start of bedtime. They are learning that this is the space where they sleep, rather than on you or with you assisting them. They are learning that you are there for them when they're upset, but that they have to put themselves to sleep.

After about 3 days your child will be used to going to sleep in this way at bedtime.

Once your child has got the hang of self-settling to sleep at bedtime, move on to the next stage of the process.

Stage Two

Voice to soothe at bedtime, halfway across the room

1. Your child should be self-settling at bedtime with you sitting next to them.
2. Now you will move to halfway across the room instead of right next to your child.
3. Continue reassuring them if they are crying with voice to soothe.
4. Overnight, put your child back to sleep using whatever method you used previously (patting, cuddling) for the time being.

   Once your child is settling better at the start of bedtime, after around 3 days, move on to the next stage of the process.

Stage Three

Voice to soothe at bedtime, at the door

1. Your child should be self-settling at bedtime with you sitting across the room from them.
2. Now you will move to the door of the room.
3. Some children might be fine with you leaving the room at this point.
4. Continue reassuring them if they are crying with voice to soothe.
5. Overnight, put your child back to sleep using whatever method you used previously (patting, cuddling) for the time being.

Stage Four

Voice to soothe at bedtime and overnight, leaving the room

1. Your child should be self-settling at bedtime with you sitting by the door.
2. Now you will leave the room.
3. Continue reassuring them if they are crying with voice

to soothe, but make sure you leave the room again each time. If you can talk to your child over your baby monitor, this is a good option.

4. From this point onward, if your child is self-settling at bedtime without you needing to use voice to soothe, they might happily self-settle overnight. If not, you can now tackle any remaining night wakes as per the instructions below.

If your child is self-settling well for bedtime without you needing to use voice to soothe AND you are not needing to stay in the room while they fall asleep, their night waking may have significantly reduced as they will be able to self-settle here too.

If, however, your child is still waking in the night you can start to respond to these wakes with voice to soothe once your child is self-settling at the start of naps and at bedtime without your help.

The method is the same as it has been previously – when your child wakes, leave them to settle themselves back to sleep. If they get upset and it's been more than 6 minutes (or a time you're comfortable with), use voice to soothe. Repeat as necessary but do not help them to sleep.

**Please note: If you are uncomfortable with any level of crying, you can soothe your child at any stage, just bear in mind the process will take longer, and you will need to be careful you're not continuing to soothe/pat/cuddle your child's to sleep long-term. You need to still be progressing through the stages.*

EARLY MORNING WAKING

If you're anything like me, 5:00 AM is not what I call morning. Early rising is a really common sleep challenge and something that can, after a while, wear pretty darn thin. Fortunately, it isn't too hard to combat the early wake, so let's have a look at how we can help with your little one being up with the larks.

Nap Structure

In this age bracket, your little one should no longer need a daytime sleep. If your child is still napping, it will most likely be the cause of that early wake and the only solution is to cut the nap altogether. Make sure you bring bedtime forwards for a while during this transition to avoid overtiredness.

Overtiredness

A child who goes to bed overtired in the evening can definitely then wake in the wee small hours and refuse to go back to sleep! To avoid overtiredness, bring bedtime forwards to between 6:00-6:30 PM.

Sleep Environment

The environment your little one sleeps in can have a huge effect on that early morning wake.

We would recommend having blackout blinds on your windows, or covering the windows with blankets to keep the light out. Between 5:00-6:00 AM sunlight can start to creep through your little one's windows and this will signal to their body clock that it is morning. If you don't want to start your day this early (and who does?!) make sure you're blocking any light from entering the room in the early hours. It's amazing the difference this small change can make.

We also strongly recommend the use of a toddler sleeping bag or sleepsack to help your little one feel snug and prevent them from getting too cold - another factor for early waking, as 5:00 AM is often the coolest part of the night.

Habit Wake

Our body clocks are truly amazing things and can be triggered by some crucial stimuli into creating a habit wake. This is likely what's happening if your toddler is waking at the exact same time each morning. It could be that they started waking early due to the factors we've listed here - overtiredness, sunlight etc, but a habit wake can very quickly form and even once the initial reason for the wake is addressed, the habit can remain.

To stop the habit waking, treat the wake like a night wake. Keep the lights off, keep communication to an absolute minimum (boring sentences like "it's sleep time") and don't engage in dialogue or a lengthy Q&A, offer water if necessary, but no calories. Your goal is to make it really unappealing for your little one to continue waking. You might have to check-in on them and repeat the boring sleep phrase several times over the course of a few nights to teach them to go back to sleep.

Sleep Training Clock Method

Another great way to tackle an early waking habit is with the aid of a sleep training clock. There are many types available and they all do the same thing – you set the clock to the time you are happy to establish as "morning" and the clock will show a different color or image when it is "morning".

You can do the same thing by using a timer device plugged into a radio or special light in your child's room. The radio/clock/light switching on will signal to your child that they are allowed to get out of bed.

This won't happen automatically. You have to retrain your child's body clock to establish the new time. If your child is waking at 5:30 AM and their new training clock isn't indicating morning until 7:00 AM they will not be able to achieve the goal of staying in their bed until morning. They are, essentially, being set up to fail.

Children are very emotionally driven – they want to do the right thing and be praised for it. Setting small achievable goals is the best way to teach them.

To do this, after explaining the concept of the training clock to your little one, you set the "morning" time on the clock to the time your child is already waking. On the first day, they will naturally wake and also see that it is morning on their clock. Goal achieved – they have stayed in their bed until "morning". Praise them!

Every 2 days you move the morning wake time on their clock back by 5 minutes. Each time, your child has to wait a little bit longer but they will know that they are able to achieve the goal. Always praise their efforts. After a while they will start naturally waking later and later as you are pushing out the times on their clock.

NIGHTMARES & NIGHT TERRORS

Children in this age bracket definitely start to have nightmares as their imagination kicks in and they're exposed more and more to external stimuli, stories, TV shows and books which can inadvertently trigger unpleasant dreams. You might notice your little one is shouting out, crying, waking afraid. Are these nightmares? Or...

Night terrors, which are a different kettle of fish. So let's explore the difference.

Night Terrors

These occur in the earlier part of the night, prior to midnight, during deep sleep. They can be more common in boys and between the ages of 2-4 years old (often linked with a surge in testosterone). Night terrors are so called because they're terrifying to witness, but your child is not actually awake during the episode (despite their eyes being open) and will have no memory of it come morning. When experiencing a night terror, children will cry, sob, shout out and may even speak coherently, but they're not awake and cannot be reasoned with. There is no evidence to suggest night terrors mean your child is terrified of something; it is thought that they are stuck between sleep cycles in a very deep sleep stage. Night terrors can be brought on by overtiredness as well as low levels of tryptophan, an enzyme that helps induce sleep. If your child is having a night terror, the best thing you can do is sit with them until it's over and tuck them back into bed afterwards. Interestingly, giving your child a banana before bed can actually help night terrors because bananas contain a lot of tryptophan! Making sure your child is having a decent/early bedtime and no sugary snacks before bed is helpful too.

Nightmares

These occur during all sleep stages, but after midnight, in your child's lighter sleep phases, they can wake your child up and are more memorable. Your child will likely wake fully after having a nightmare and can be consoled and taken back to bed, usually with full memory of the incident the next day. Nightmares begin once children have developed active imagination - somewhere beyond 2 years old. Until your child understands the mature concept of fear, they will not be having nightmares as we know them. For babies or younger toddlers who are whimpering or crying in their sleep, or waking upset, this is usually attributed to other factors such as being too hot or cold, being sick, trapped wind, uncomfortable digestion, overtiredness inhibiting deep sleep, or other more serious factors like reflux.

Some tips to help with nightmares:

- Ensure your child isn't exposed to anything on TV or in books or games that is scary!
- Have a decent, calm wind-down time before bed with no screens and no sugary foods or drinks
- Make sure your child's bedtime stories are gentle and not too stimulating or frightening (no dragons or monsters!)
- Giving your child foods that are high in tryptophan during the day can lead to more restful sleep - some examples are sour cherries, bananas, turkey, dairy foods
- Ensure your little one isn't overtired at bedtime. Aim for a day of no longer than 13 hours for them, from wake-up in the morning until bedtime at night.

Nightmares (especially ongoing nightmares) in children can sometimes lead to bed or room aversion, where they associate their bed or their room with being afraid. If this starts to happen to your little one, make sure you read our section on bed/room aversion for the best way to tackle this.

BEDWETTING & NIGHT TOILET TRAINING

Between the ages of 3-6 years old, most children will be working on night toilet training. This can come with its own set of challenges. Even once your child is toilet trained at night, there can definitely still be bouts of bedwetting and in some cases, this can continue into their school years.

Firstly, let's look at night training:

Night training your child can come anytime from 2 weeks to a year after they are day trained. Your child absolutely has to take the lead on this one. Your indicators are very simple and will be:

- your child wakes with a dry night nappy/diaper every morning for 2 weeks
- your child suddenly starts sleeping worse in the night; waking for no apparent reason (they may or may not have a dry nappy/diaper in the morning). This is a tricky one to pinpoint as night waking can also be due to many other factors. Usually if your child has been day-trained for quite a while and you can rule out sickness or any other factor, they are probably waking because their body is telling them they need to pee but they haven't yet learnt how to deal with going pee in the night. They will then not be able to easily go back to sleep because they have a full bladder and don't want to consciously go pee in their nappy.

Night training is extremely simple. If your child has been waking in the morning for 2 weeks with a consistently dry nappy/diaper, your work is done! Make sure your child always goes pee before bed and has no liquids to drink in the hour leading up to bedtime. Discuss with them that they don't need their night diaper anymore, but don't use underwear on them at night for the first few weeks – just loose pajama pants. (Having tight clothes around their bottom might make the child feel they're in a nappy/diaper again and they might have some accidents.) We would recommend having a waterproof mattress cover on your child's bed.

If you are in the second group and your child has started waking because they need to pee, it will take a little more effort to train them at night. The method is similar to dream feeding a baby, however you are "dream pottying" your child – taking them pee in the night without them really fully waking. Still explain to your child that they don't need their night diaper/nappy anymore and also reinforce that it's ok for them to wake and go pee in the potty/toilet during the night. Sometimes just explaining this is enough for them to night train.

To "dream-potty" your child, just before you go to bed take the potty into their room, get them gently out of their bed and sit them on the potty. Tell them to go pee (you might need to repeat this a few times). Be patient. After they go, put them back in bed. Repeat this for a few nights until they either refuse to go, or the quantity of their pee is much reduced, or they are confident waking on their own for a pee. They are learning to control their bladder at night by learning to wake to go to the toilet. It does help to vary the times you get them up as they may start to develop a habit of needing to pee at that time if it continues for an extended period. Most children will, after a couple of nights, simply refuse to go when you wake them, however just getting them used to the idea of waking at night if they need to pee will generally ensure they start sleeping a lot better.

There may be a few bed wettings, but if your child is good and ready to train at night you might not encounter any at all. Make sure you praise them and reinforce their good night toileting habits in the morning.

If a week has passed of getting them up at night and they are still peeing good quantities during the night, firstly limit their fluid intake significantly before bed (if your child is still having a bottle of milk at bedtime, it's probably time to reduce then stop this). If they continue to pee a lot overnight they might not be quite ready to night train yet. You are better to wait until they have had 2 weeks of consistently dry nappies/diapers in the morning.

Always make sure your child goes pee as soon as they wake in the morning and keep reinforcing their amazing efforts!

Bedwetting

In this section we're going to look at bedwetting that occurs once your child has already been night toilet trained for over 6 months. Bedwetting is quite common in children and affects approximately:

- 15 percent of 5 year olds
- 5 percent of 10 year olds
- 2 percent of 15 year olds

Bedwetting generally presents as a child who, on relatively regular occasions, wakes in the night having wet their bed; we're not talking about those random occurrences every now and then, that can happen to almost every child at some point. The first and most important thing to remember is that they have not done this on purpose or to be naughty, and as frustrating and tiring as bedwetting can be for a parent, we need to remain calm and approach this issue with kindness and understanding. The other key thing to remember is that most children do eventually grow out of bedwetting - there is an end in sight!

There are several causes of bedwetting in children:

- Their waking response to a full bladder overnight hasn't fully developed yet
- Your child's bladder cannot hold the amount of pee they produce overnight
- Constipation
- Your child has an overactive bladder, which also means they likely have accidents during the day too or have sudden urgent needs to pee in the day
- Less commonly, bedwetting can be due to a urinary tract infection (UTI), increased anxiety, or stress (such as a new sibling, starting daycare etc)

Whatever you think the cause of bedwetting is for your child, here are some tips to work through this issue:

1. As we mentioned, keep calm and respond gently when your child wets the bed. You don't want to make it a big issue that could turn into a point of anxiety or embarrassment for your child.
2. Lots of positive reinforcement and praise when your child gets up at night to use the toilet.
3. Have a nightlight in your child's room and/or the toilet - in some cases, children with a fear of the dark simply do not want to get out of bed on their own to go to the toilet in the dark.
4. Give your child lots of fluids during the day (but not in the hour before bedtime), to train their bladder to hold more fluids.
5. Make sure your child goes to the toilet and does a pee before bedtime - however long it takes.
6. If you are dream-toileting your child (as per our night toilet training method), make sure your child is fully awake and aware of going to the toilet.
7. Use a waterproof mattress protector to save your

bedding if bedwetting is a regular occurrence in your house. This makes those middle of the night bed changes a lot easier.

8. Regular bedwetting isn't considered a problem by experts until your little one is over 7 years old. Most of these strategies will put a stop to bedwetting prior to that.
9. Do not put nappies/diapers on children over 4 as it can lead to anxiety and embarrassment

If you're worried about your child's bedwetting, experts recommend seeking help from a medical professional if your child has been dry at night for over a year and suddenly starts bedwetting, or if they are still bedwetting regularly over the age of 7, or if the bedwetting (at any age) is causing problems within your family.

SHARING A ROOM WITH A SIBLING

Whether out of necessity or preference, chances are that your little ones will, at some point, have to share a room. Even if it's just while you're on vacation or for a short time. This doesn't have to be as stressful as it sounds!

In most scenarios the best advice we can give you is to always put the youngest child to bed first. This works well for two main reasons:

1. The littlest will generally be the most tired and can't hold out for a slightly later bedtime (and an overtired baby or toddler is no one's friend).
2. The older child will have more understanding of the need to be quieter and more respectful of their little sleeping sibling.

The exception to this rule is if you have a baby under 6 months old who is still on 3 naps a day. In this case, you can shift their daytime schedule backwards by say half an hour, or let them nap for slightly longer in the last nap, so that they can aim for a slightly later bedtime. This means you can put your tired older child to bed first, then your baby about half an hour after that. Your older child should be good and tired and will be deeply asleep by the time the baby is going to bed. Once, however, your baby is down to just 2 naps a day, you'll probably want to put them to bed first to avoid overtiredness.

Here are our expert tips to make room sharing a lot easier:

- Use white noise all night long. Not only will this help your little ones sleep better, it'll also mask any sounds either child might make in the night, including sleep talking, getting up to use the bathroom, snoring, teeth grinding.

- Do the bedtime routine for each child outside of the bedroom (stories, songs etc). This means that they can go into bed sleepy and ready for bed (meaning they'll settle quicker), and you won't risk waking the already-sleeping child with stories for the older one.

- If you're in the throes of sleep training your littler one, perhaps put the older child in a different room (or your room) for a few nights so they're not woken by their sibling.

- Give each child their own "space" in the room so they have specific areas they can call their own. This will make them feel more comfortable about sharing a room - especially if they're a bit older, or if one child is moving into the other child's room.

- Be patient! Moves like this are a really massive deal to our little ones and there can definitely be some ups and downs during the adjustment period. Staying calm and being tolerant and respectful of the big change is really key to helping your children adapt to this new normal.

SCREENS & SLEEP

There is a lot of controversy and opinions out there regarding how much (if any) screen time children should be having and we're not going to weigh in on screen time in a general sense. But, whether you're for or against your little ones watching TV, there is still an area most experts agree should be off-limits... screens before bed.

Here's why:

In the evening, our bodies are gearing up for sleep. This means a bunch of amazing processes are kicking off to help us fall asleep and stay asleep when bedtime comes around. Hormones like melatonin are crucial to this process and this particular hormone is produced in response to diminishing light in the evening. Now, in this modern world, we don't really let the light diminish as naturally as it should in the lead-up to bedtime, so this process is automatically a bit harder for our bodies. But when you throw in exposure to blue/white light (which is the light emitted from TVs and screens), you're really starting to mess with the biological process of sleep.

Blue light is the worst type of light when it comes to sleep. This light mimics bright daylight more closely than any other coloured light and will trick our bodies into thinking it's still the middle of the day. You can see how this would interrupt the sleep process. When our children (and also ourselves) are exposed to this harsh light right before bedtime, it's really inhibiting the release of those crucial sleep hormones, which will lead to more difficulty with settling and also a more restless sleep.

Another factor to consider about screens/TV before bed, is the affect the content can have on your little one's sleep. These days TV shows and games on iPads/phones are very stimulating in terms of their graphics and also their content. To unwind from this, it can take quite a process for our children to switch their brains off from the extreme stimulation and engaging story content.

Screens before bed are not going to help your children settle and sleep.

We would recommend:

- Having a screens-off policy 2 hours before bedtime (this includes TVs, iPads/tablets, phones)
- Dimming the lights in your house (or turning some off) 1 hour before bedtime
- Doing quiet activities in the lead-up to bedtime, these could include
    - Reading stories
    - Doing puzzles
    - Listening to music
    - Lego or building blocks
    - Talking or singing
    - Mindfulness or meditation
    - Audiobooks

SECTION 2:

Behavior

TANTRUMS & HOW TO DEAL WITH THEM

Why Do Kids Have Tantrums?

It's safe to say that all parents are familiar with tantrums. Whether we like it or not, these "meltdowns", which typically occur between 1-4 years of age, are a part of healthy toddler and childhood development. As adults, we have had many years to cultivate a range of different coping techniques to help us manage the demands of day to day life, but our kids have not yet had the chance to develop these skills. Tantrums are a child's way of telling us that they don't know how to cope with whatever situation they are in, and they are not at all happy about it! Often a tantrum is a response to being told "no", having to complete a task they don't want to do, ending a task they are currently enjoying, or perhaps it's because we have removed them from a dangerous situation. My toddler currently enjoys jumping off of things. Usually this is fine; it's great to be active, he's developing spatial awareness and gross motor skills, but when it's not safe and he is physically removed, of course he protests...loudly!

Tantrums (and lying, as language develops) are also a child's ways of testing boundaries and learning about manipulation. Rest assured that there is rarely any malicious intent, but kids are inherently selfish and want what they want. They haven't yet learned how to put themselves in another person's shoes, to think logically when they're emotional, and empathize with others. They don't know how to negotiate, to delay gratification, and effectively manage frustrations. They want what they want, and aren't scared to have a public meltdown to get what they want (their determination is actually quite admirable!) As our kids are trying to work out how to get their way, as parents, we are often the guinea pigs they can road-test these new skills on. This is why sometimes our kids are better behaved with others than they are when they are with us. They know we love them unconditionally, and they may take advantage of that. Annoying but normal and often a sign of a strong, secure attachment.

Tantrums can also become quite common as your child starts to become more independent. In these cases, tantrums are their way of communicating with us that they want to do something, and often in a certain way, so much so that if you help them, they may become upset. Tantrums are also common when kids are tired, hungry, or unwell...and let's be honest, this doesn't change even in adulthood!

But wait, there's more!

Sometimes there is just too much happening, which can be draining on your toddler's senses as they try to process things. Their mind may be in overdrive trying to make sense of the situation, but can't keep up! This will often happen in public places where there are lots of people and noises, like a party. They're trying to process all the different faces, noises, conversations, smells, movements, and objects. To help you understand what it could be like, imagine going to sleep and then opening your eyes and suddenly, you're in a foreign country.

You don't speak the language well, you aren't sure where you are, everything looks different. It's bright, crowded, and loud. It's a bit overwhelming, maybe scary, and you need a few minutes to get your head around it all or need some comfort. This is why your little one may be clinging to you, or may cry initially.

So...what can you do to help?

First things first, we need to identify the function of the tantrum or understand why it's occurring. What are our kids trying to communicate with us? The reason for the tantrum will often determine how we can best respond and manage their distress.

They're testing boundaries and flexing their desire for control: When our kids are testing boundaries and have a tantrum to try to get a response from us, you'll usually see a couple of things: 1) They place themselves down on the ground either gently or very dramatically; and 2) they will often check to ensure that we are paying attention to them. They may look up every now and then to see if we are watching. After all, a tantrum to get their way doesn't work if we aren't there to receive the message hidden in the tantrum. If you see this happening, you are welcome to reason with your children once, using limited language (avoid a long speech). Something brief which acknowledges their distress, but sets a firm boundary. For example, *"I know you're upset, you want to play, but we need to tidy up first"*. As they continue to tantrum, you can simply reiterate your point, again briefly, but then you may need to sit back and let them go through the emotional roller-coaster. Try not to cave in! Be present, express empathy, but be firm in your decision. When they eventually calm down, give them a cuddle, get on with the task, and afterwards, reiterate that now it's time for them to have what they want. In this instance, you could say *"We have tidied up, thank-you for your help! Now let's play!"*

If your little one escalates and you can see that they have become completely overwhelmed by their emotions, we need to slow down and reconnect before we can redirect or apply logic. This is also helpful if they are overloaded by their environment. A child who is having an emotional meltdown will not be able to respond to anything reasonable or logical you have to say if they're emotionally overwhelmed. When these tantrums occur, they will continue wailing whether you are there or not, they're inconsolable, and you can see they are beyond the point of having any control over themselves. We may also notice ourselves feeling upset with them, rather than frustrated. When this occurs, we need to lower our own energy, our voice, and our height, and sometimes move them to a different space which will help lower their level of distress. Speak slowly, softly, validate their experience, and simply be available and present. You can even offer a cuddle. If they don't want a cuddle, that's okay. Maybe offer a few words of comfort here and there, but if the tantrum seems to be due to overload, the less input you give for them to process, the better. It will pass if you give them the time and space they need.

They're upset because of a "No" or they can't have what they want: Kids will quickly develop an aversion to "no". It seems so final to our little ones! That in mind, it can be helpful to use a different word. Sometimes "no" really means "it's not safe", or "later, but not right now". Try changing the words you use and help kids focus on what they can do, or what you want them to do, rather than what not to do. For example, if you're walking together, instead of saying *"don't walk on the road"*, ask them to *"walk on the footpath"*. If they ignore you, repeat yourself, ensuring you have their attention by making eye contact. If their behavior is not safe (e.g. walking on the road) let them know with a short instruction.

Something like *"it's not safe to walk there, we need to walk here"*, and gently move them onto the footpath. If they accept this, show your child you're proud of them, and maybe offer a reward (but be sure to keep rewards spontaneous, we want to avoid kids only engaging in positive behavior when there is a reward). If a tantrum ensues, know that they are testing boundaries, which you know how to manage. To help satisfy their need for control and making decisions, forced choice can also be helpful. This is when you give them 2-3 options that you're happy for them to select from. When we do this, they get to make a decision, but within your boundaries. For example, instead of saying *"We can't go to the park because it's raining"*, try *"When it stops raining, we can go outside. But right now, we can either bake cookies or read. What would you like to do right now?"*

Take time for you!

Sometimes we manage tantrums well and can shake it off. Other times, they really get under our skin and we feel like boiling over. If you're at the point where you feel a tantrum of your own coming on, remove yourself from the situation. Ensure your little one is safe, and go into a different room to reset. It's hard to support a little one through a tantrum when we're at breaking point ourselves. You also need to invest in your own well-being – raising kids is hard! I recommend trying to find at least 30 minutes every day to focus on yourself. We've all heard the saying "you can't pour from an empty cup", and it's so true! If Mamma is unhappy, the kids will pick up on it. Be sure to take care of you! In fact, I challenge you all to create a self-care calendar whereby every day, you roster in a 30 minutes self-care activity.

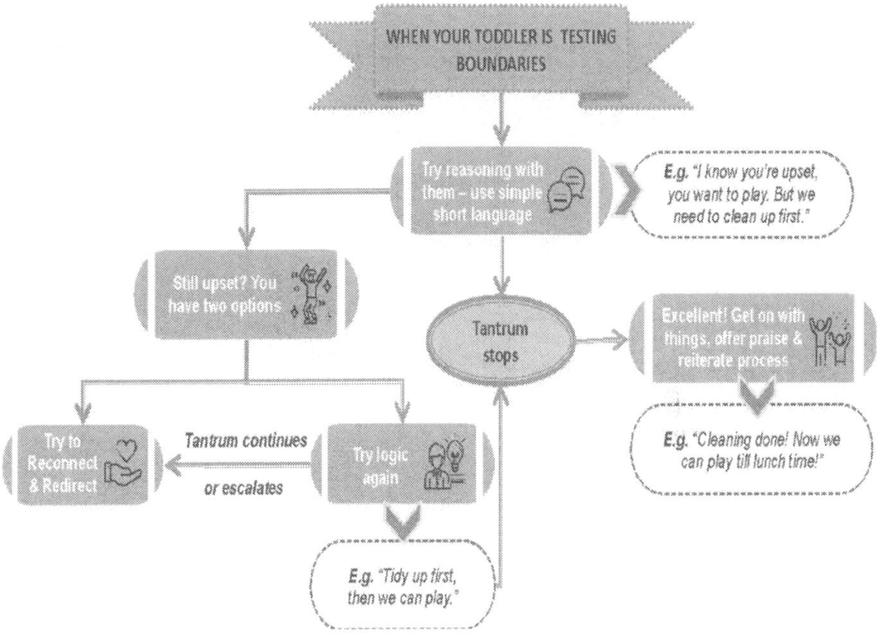

If you are feeling really overwhelmed, why not speak to a professional? Have a chat with your GP and discuss your referral options. There are many healthcare professionals here to help, such as Pediatricians, Psychologists, Psychiatrists, and Occupational Therapists. You don't have to do it alone!

Reconnect and Redirect when your little one is overwhelmed

1. Lower yourself to their level physically, speak softly, slowly and calmly. If you're in a public place, try to find somewhere quieter or less busy.
2. Validate their experience e.g. *"This is really upsetting for you. It's okay to feel upset"*...then wait.
3. Just be present, supportive and calm. If you notice a subtle de-escalation in the tantrum, you can validate again, offer a drink, or a cuddle. Otherwise, simply wait and ensure your little one has the safe space they need to regain control of their emotions.
4. Once the tantrum subsides, recognise this and provide encouragement e.g. *"That was so hard for you, but you got through it. I'm proud of you"*.

If your little one becomes upset when you say "No"

1. Use different words, such as *"We can do that later"* or *"It's not safe to do that."*
2. Focus on what they can do and what you want e.g. *"We need to walk on the footpath where it's safer."*
3. Use forced choice and give 2-3 options you are happy with them to choose from e.g. *"You can read some books, or we can make some cookies. What would you prefer?"*

You can combine these techniques! For example, if your little one is upset because it's raining and they want to go outside, you could say "*We can go outside when it stops raining. For now, we can read or bake cookies! What do you want to do?*"

Please note, if your toddler is being unsafe, you need to take action! Physically move them into a safe place. If a tantrum occurs, go back to the flow chart on managing tantrums when your toddler is testing boundaries.

DEALING WITH A NEW SIBLING OR A BIG CHANGE

Big life changes are inevitable and are a normal part of life, and as such we can prepare ourselves or recover after the change. That being said, we still might not like change or find it particularly easy to cope with. Although we can understand it as adults, our children find change incredibly challenging and even scary at times, even if the change seems to be a positive or exciting one. Changes are scary for children because they don't understand necessarily why it happens (or cannot make sense of the change), they often aren't involved in discussions or choices that result in change (so they feel insignificant and disempowered) but more importantly our children haven't fully developed their capacity to regulate their emotions and are still building their resilience, both of which help our children respond to and bounce back from diversity.

Throughout our lives we face challenges and develop resilience incrementally with each problem we face. For each hurdle we jump over we find new ways of managing and coping; however, our children are still young, with very limited life experience to draw from which means that they need additional support to manage their big feelings and increased compassion and understanding when they are adjusting to changes.

What are some of the big changes that might impact our

children?

Because our children are so little, we need to consider that any change could be a big change. They tend to have very little say in what happens in their world, and are also still learning how their world and the people in it work. So, because they don't have this context they can struggle with even small changes like transitioning between activities or a change in season that results in an appropriate change in wardrobe/outfit selections.

Some of the key, and bigger changes that may be normal/ appropriate during childhood (the list is by no means exhaustive), but which our little people struggle with could be;

- Birth of a sibling – having to share parental or familial attention, perhaps a change in room to accommodate the baby, reduction or cessation in breastfeeding, change in mum's body, having higher expectations on them once their sibling is born, developing a new relationship with their sibling. New babies can also result in changes to parent/caregiver's work circumstances which may impact on increased or decreased presence of parents, potential impacts on finances and even added strain or stress that comes with welcoming a new baby into the family. Even older children can struggle with these changes, it's not only toddlers and young children who can find it hard to accept the changes associated with a new sibling.

- Starting formal care or school and also changing carers/ school – whether that be school or childcare, or even a shared caregiving arrangement with friends/family etc. Any big change in routine can be challenging for our children to manage, but having to adapt to adhering to someone else's routine, or being one in a group can be particularly hard. They also need to learn about the new people caring for them and they can potentially feel unsafe whilst they figure out the new "rules" and expectations the person or people have.

- Moving house or relocating (for family, health or jobs etc) – can be a really confusing time for children, in their early years their house is pretty much their whole world. They can get distressed at leaving somewhere familiar, in particular if they are also moving away from family, friends or neighbors they have known for a long time. It's also the familiarity of the house itself (the building) and memories or routines they developed in the house that can be challenging to transition away from.

- Death of a family member or pet – we all learn about grief and loss at some point in our lives, but for children (depending on their age) the permanency of the loss might not sink in for a really long time, particularly for younger children who are still coming to terms with "object permanence" (the idea that objects continue to exist despite not being seen/heard/sensed). This can make the adjustment to life without the person (or even their pet) hard, because they may not understand they have died and may relive their grief multiple times, or they may have limited emotional response at all because they don't truly understand where their loved one has gone and why (lack of emotional response can sometimes be harder for parents to deal with).

- Parents/caregivers separating – even if the separation is amicable, children have to readjust to having two homes, or not seeing a primary caregiver 100% of the time. Without the same routines or rules, they can struggle to feel safe and secure because everything is new, and the issue of object permanence might come up again, they may not be able to understand where their caregiver has gone (if there is no shared custody). Separation may also mean a change in home/living circumstances/school/finances alongside the change in caregiving which is a lot for even us adults to adjust to.

- Illness – whether it be illness of the child or a significant person in their life, illness can radically shift the daily life of families. New routines to manage the health issue, changes in capacity of parents to give undivided attention, separation (if the person has to move for treatment or attended extended hospital stays). The child may also not yet have the developmental capacity to understand about the illness itself and how symptoms manifest or what treatment is required, not all children should be given this level of information (it may or may not be appropriate depending on their cognitive capacity), but without context or rational as to why big changes are occurring their lives it can be hard for children to make sense of what's happening around them. They will however, be attuned to the emotions of their caregivers and will certainly know that something is wrong/different/worrying and can still pick up and respond strongly despite not even being aware that a loved one is unwell.

HOW DO CHILDREN RESPOND TO CHANGE?

Developmentally our young children are working hard to make sense of the world around them. They rely on predictability, including how the adults around them will behave and respond to them in order to feel emotionally safe and secure. It takes a lot of energy for our children to try and figure out the context of why the change has happened and also the new "rules". Feeling unsafe or unsure can also result in emotional and behavioral changes in our children whilst they navigate the new normal.

Emotional changes

Tantrums – sometimes our children let us know (loudly) that there has been some kind of change or disruption to their equilibrium. A tantrum is an external demonstration (of disorganized behavior) that represents internal distress. You might notice behaviors such as; crying, shouting, a stiff or arching body, kicking/punching/flailing, self-injurious behavior (hair pulling, head banging, scratching), fleeing/running away or even vomiting and holding their breath.

Tantrums most commonly occur between the ages of one and four, but during periods of distress or adjustment it is normal to see tantrums in much older children. They generally occur because our children are struggling to make sense of their big emotions or have become so overwhelmed, they have lost control. This loss of control (or perceived loss of control, including emotional overwhelm) can result in a tantrum because it might be the only way our children can express frustration or distress over a change that doesn't make sense to them. Having a tantrum might also be the only way your child knows how to bring back control over their environment and the people in it.

Personality/emotional changes – you may notice a marked shift in your child's usual personality or emotional expression. They may have previously been bubbly and boisterous, and now they are quiet and withdrawn, or perhaps your child was reserved and now they are vocal and possibly disruptive. What matters here is that their emotional response to the world has shifted from what you consider the "norm" for your child. Marked changes in mood is something you might want to consider seeking support for, with a trusted health professional. Another change to be aware of is clinginess or reduced independence, if your child is feeling unsure or unsafe due to changes, they may be more reliant on their caregiver to regulate their emotions or to anchor them. Children may become clingy to elicit more attention and time with a carer, they could be struggling with separation or transitioning between care (i.e. home and school) and/or between activities.

Behavioral changes

Limit testing – all children test limits, that's not uncommon however after a big change you may notice your child really pushing the boundaries. Generally, this occurs because they are trying to figure out a new situation; what do I do here? Do people still expect the same thing of me? What's the same and what's different than before? Limit testing can also arise if our kids notice we are more lenient or distracted. After a big change if our children are distressed and overwhelmed it can be tempting to let things slide because we empathize with their upset, or potentially the change has had a big impact on us as adults and it's harder/

exhausting to uphold previous rules/limits. A limit helps a child know what to expect from a person or situation so they feel more secure and confident to manage, because they know what will happen. However, if we aren't consistent with our limits it can inadvertently make things worse as our children feel even more unsafe. Kids don't necessarily like limits, but they do need them because they make them feel safe and cared for.

Regression – after a period of stress or change children's behavior and development may regress. Regression refers to the loss of skills which were recently acquired or they may even move backwards in terms of their development. We see this often in toileting, sleeping or returning to a stage requiring self-nurturing or nurturing from a caregiver, things like; sucking thumbs, babbling, wanting to be fed or carried like a baby. In the vast majority of cases once the stressor or situation has settled most children re-learn or revert back to a mature stage of development. However, in childhood there are developmental disorders which do need to be investigated; you know your child and your family the best. So, this is another situation where you may want to see the support of a trusted health professional if your child's regression is not linked to a big change/stressful event or doesn't improve after things settle down.

Changes to eating/sleeping patterns – one key marker of changes to mental health/wellbeing is someone's eating or sleeping patterns. This could be considered to be emotional or behavioral, but will be included under the banner of "behavioral" as what parents notice is the outward expression of their child's distress. Low mood, stress and anxiety can all impact on our sleeping and eating patterns, whether it be eating/sleeping too much, or the opposite not wanting (or not being able to) eat or sleep well. This relationship also goes both ways, lack of or too much sleep/food can also negatively impact on emotional and physical wellbeing. There is still a lot of research as to why sleep and eating are affected, but simplistically it is thought to come down to hormones being released in the body or changes to brain waves/patterns and other physiological changes associated with stress, anxiety and other mood disorders. In regards to eating, there is another element potentially at play here. Our children often do not have a lot of control over things in their lives, but what they eat and how much they eat is one area where they can make choices and decisions. If your child's world is feeling out of control, they may start to focus on areas of their lives that they can control. It is normal in the aftermath of a stressful event or disruption to notice some changes to eating and sleeping, but they are also something to watch very carefully and seek support with if you notice markedly different or prolonged changes, and you see things like loss of weight, reduced energy, trouble concentrating.

SUPPORTING YOUR CHILD TO MANAGE CHANGE

It is important to know that managing change is tough at any age, and we cannot take away the distress or discomfort of this from our children. But we do need to help them learn how to cope, so that next time change occurs, and every time after, that they are more prepared and increasingly better able to manage all of the challenges that come with big changes.

Name the feeling and give it context

When we don't understand what is happening to us or why it can add to the feeling of overwhelm and confusion. Our children have to learn about their feelings in the same way they learn about anything else...from us teaching them. When they are infants' they see a cat, and we name it *"See that cat, isn't it cute?"* We then help them to compare and contrast so they understand the difference between say a cat and a turtle *"Cats have fur, pointy ears, whiskers and tails. Turtles have a hard shell and flippers"*.

We then also teach our kids about the different variations so they can understand that although they might see lots of cats' they may have different variations; grey cats, furless cats, fluffy cats, big cats etc. This is exactly the same for emotions, we need to teach our kids to know the different names of their feelings and be able to identify them, understand how they differ from other feelings and also know that there are different variations of an individual feeling, for example; anger can range from mere frustration right through to red hot rage.

- *"I can see you feel angry right now because your sister didn't share her toy."*
- *"It seems like you are a bit sad. I wonder if it's because you miss your granny?"*

Our children also need to understand how their feelings connect with their experiences so they can understand their world better and can then prepare themselves or implement coping strategies. When it comes to big changes our children can often feel out of control of the situation, so if we can offer them knowledge and context around their emotional response to the change, they can feel more in control of one area of their lives when all else feels confusing.

It might also be helpful to help your child understand that excitement and nervousness often feel the same. Butterflies in the tummy, sweating or shaking and also thinking about the upcoming event a lot can be explained by nerves/worry as well as excitement. You might want to talk to them about the different feelings in their body as well as the idea that even though change might be worrying, the result could be something exciting or positive. Not all changes have to be bad, but we still need to acknowledge the impact of upheaval and change in itself being disruptive.

Normalize

It's ok to have big feelings and it's ok for your child to struggle or feel overwhelmed at times. They may experience grief and loss associated with the change and what their life used to be like "before". When we normalize, we don't rush our children through their feelings, or try to convince them that their feelings aren't valid.

Normalizing is simply accepting their feelings as they exist and helps them to feel seen and acknowledged.

- Imagine one day you wake up late because the alarm doesn't go off, then you make a coffee and realize the milk is off, then your child misplaces their shoes and you can't find their sports uniform, then as you head out of the house you accidentally lock your keys (car keys included) in the house. What if you called a friend to vent about your day and they said "It's not that bad, don't worry, there's no need to complain about it." You would feel pretty upset that they weren't being supportive. You didn't ask them to make your day better or try and change it, but they didn't even hear you or acknowledge how your day had been! However, imagine that they responded in a different way *"Oh my gosh that sounds like such a tough day and I completely understand how challenging it was, I bet you were so frustrated!"* You would feel really different and that's the power of normalizing. Sometimes you don't need to fix things, you just need to be present and help your child know that it's normal to feel scared/angry/sad etc about changes.

Modeling

Acknowledge your own emotional response, and thoughts around the change (in a developmentally appropriate way of course) with your child. It can be tempting to try and protect our kids from being affected by change, or many can feel that pressure to be a perfect parent who is coping. It generally comes from a protective place because parents don't want their children to get worried or feel responsible for their parents' distress; however, our children will notice those emotional changes in their parents anyway. If we don't give our children some context (again developmentally appropriate levels of sharing) then they use their imagination to put all the missing pieces together, and what they imagine is often much worse than the reality, and it can often include self-blame. Children are egocentric (focussed on themselves) so they will often focus their thoughts back onto themselves. By acknowledging our feelings and thoughts about change, parents are not only helping their children to make sense of the change, but it's also a good opportunity to model and explore coping strategies.

- *"I'm feeling nervous about moving to a new house. I love our house now and it's so close to your aunt's house and cousins so I'm worried about whether I will like this new house as much. It's really normal to feel worried about change, so I'm going to write down the things I'm excited about for this new house so I remember some of the good stuff too!"*
- *"I feel a bit scared about my new job because I won't know anyone there. I wonder if you feel worried too about meeting new friends at school? Let's think of some ways together to try and feel better. Maybe we can plan what we might say on our first days at work and school? Or maybe we can make some plans for the weekend to catch up with family or friends so we remember that not everything and everyone has changed? What do you think?"*

Warning

Give your child as much advanced warning as you can to prepare them for a change. Of course, this is not always possible (not all changes are predictable or set in motion intentionally), and it's not always appropriate to tell very young children too far in advance as they don't always understand timeframes ("tomorrow" versus "next week" or even "in a year' time") so it can be tricky balance. Warning in advance will help your child come to terms with the upcoming changes. It doesn't mean that they will still enjoy or be ok with the change, but if they know what is happening, they will feel more in control of the event and you can help prepare them by understanding which feelings come up as you talk about the upcoming change.

- Firstly, consider if your child can understand the concept of time and decide how far in advance you can warn them and how you might help them mark the passage of time. You could set a timer (if the change is occurring within a short period of time – within the day or even hour). If the change is happening a little further down the track consider setting up a calendar on the fridge so you can mark down the days together.

- Talk about the change and steps or markers that will let them know the change is coming to better prepare them. For example; if you are moving house. You might tell your child the reason for moving, and that soon you will be looking for a new house to live in. Where possible (and appropriate) you could take them house hunting or show them pictures. You might do a drive by the new place or show them their new neighborhood, if that's not possible do some internet research and show them some pictures (particularly if your partner has had to go ahead or perhaps you are moving across the country or internationally). Let them know that soon you will be packing up your belongings so they are prepared, but give them a choice of a few things to keep in a special bag they can access. You might then let them know about what moving day might look like or help them to plan where things will go in their new room. Whatever the change, giving them information to help them understand what they need to prepare for is crucial in adjustment.

Resources

See if you can find a book or tv show which addresses the change you will soon be facing. Finding a child character of a similar age will be the most helpful as they will more readily identify with and contextualize the story if they see themselves as similar to the character. Reading a story or watching a show about a similar topic (divorce, welcoming a new sibling, a health diagnosis etc) will allow for some important teachings that as parents we can't impart so easily. Seeing a character, they connect with going through a similar process or situation and seeing them coping or managing will really normalize their feelings and help them to feel capable, hopeful and builds their resilience.

Listen

You shouldn't and cannot always fix things for your child, sometimes things are tough and we need to learn to sit with discomfort of things being out of control and resulting in big feelings. Instead of rushing to try and sort things out so that your child doesn't feel distressed about a change, spend some time listening to them. The act of listening and empathizing is so impactful because the person genuinely feels heard, respected and sometimes when we rush to fix a problem, we accidentally undermine how big or impactful it feels for the person. So sometimes just listening can be the most powerful way of supporting your child (or anyone) through a big emotion or change.

- To actively listen; get on your child level and make eye contact, have open and relaxed body posture and angle your body towards them...this is showing that you are really listening and engaged with what they are saying based on the signals of your body.
- Dedicate some protected time. Don't ask your child important questions or bring up big topics when you are in the middle of homework/dinner prep/doing the laundry. Give them your undivided attention and plan in some time for just the two of you to talk.
- Try not to do too much talking, ask questions and then really listen to the answer. We demonstrate good listening by asking questions (relevant to the conversation) and by reflecting back what we hear and naming any emotions we can detect *"Ahh, I understand now. You're telling me you are worried about starting school in case you don't make any friends. I can hear that is making*

you feel nervous".

Routines

When their world is changing around them, really try to keep their routines as stable as possible because structure feels safe for our children. Or if you know a change is coming up in the future, work on implementing a routine in the build-up to give them something safe and consistent to anchor them. Routines could be things that occur each day, or they could be longer term weekly/monthly routines, in particular routines that involve connection with your child are ones to really firm up and hold tight to.

- Consider your bedtime routines, can you keep the same steps; bath, brush teeth, dress into pjs, read a story together and have a cuddle. Think about the same for morning and getting ready routines. Keeping things consistent also reduces some of the pressure/stress of daily activities like the school run, or homework time etc.
- Think about family routines and your weekends or after school/work. If your child attends weekly swimming classes but you are moving house could you sign them up to the same day and similar time for swim classes near the new house? If you always visit the library on a Thursday could you go online and watch a youtuber reading a children's story, or find a new local library? Or you have play dates with their cousins on the weekend, could you replace it with a skype call to still connect at the same time?
- Increase expectations and clarity by mapping either daily routines or weekly routines/appointments on a calendar or a list of steps on a piece of paper (images instead of words works well for younger children) and hang it somewhere prominent like on the fridge or your child's bedroom door.
- You could also involve them in creating new rituals

that get them excited about the change (and see it in a positive light). For example, Fridays could become family movie nights, or on Saturdays you always go out for a family walk. It doesn't really matter what it is (but try to keep the focus on activities that involve family time or connectedness), but you can involve them in decision making about what new ritual you could introduce so that they feel more in control of things.

Give them control

Don't hand over the reins entirely, but give them more say in age appropriate decisions. When we give children control over some elements of their life, they will feel increased self-esteem and confidence in their own ability to cope, as well as their capacity to make decisions about their life. For young children it could be as simple as giving them a choice about what breakfast they eat (from a variety of appropriate options) or what clothes they wear that day or even getting them to help meal plan for the week. If your child feels in control of their everyday life then then the impact associated with change will feel less dramatic as they haven't lost control over all of the things in their life. When we allow our children to make choices and involve them in decision making it gives them a sense of agency, as well as improved self-esteem associated with seeing themselves as capable and will build their resilience and capacity to cope with changes.

Answer their questions (appropriate to their developmental level)

Sometimes change is scarier for our children when their imagination fills in the blanks, for example in cases of separation children often wonder what they did wrong that caused their caregivers to split up. We know as adults that it's nothing to do with our children, but something much bigger in the relationship, but our children are egocentric (focussed on themselves) and will often interpret changes as occurring because of them in some way. It's not to say that children need to be told about all of the nitty gritty details of a change and why it needs to happen, but they certainly need enough context to not have to use their imaginations to make sense of the situation.

- Consider the age of your child and their emotional/ cognitive maturity when you think about how much you should share. Very young children don't need to know exact details but you might tell them what changes they might notice, and why the change is occurring. For example; illness and death. You might share that a relative is experiencing a health issue (such as cancer) and what your child might notice, but spare them some of the details *"Your aunty has been feeling unwell and she went to her doctor. They said she needs to take some medicine that might make her feel worse before she starts to feel better. You might notice that she can't do the same things she used to as she needs to sit and lay down to rest and let her body get better."*
- Invite them to tell you what they already know about a situation. This will help you to figure out whether they have made any (incorrect) assumptions or guesses that you need to address, but also it gives you an idea about which "blanks" you might need to fill to complete their understanding of the issue.
- Encourage them to ask lots of questions, but be reassured that it's ok if you don't know the answer, maybe you need to prepare yourself with an answer before you get back to them or you could even suggest researching an answer together to find out more. *"That's a really good question, and I want to answer it, I'm just not quite sure of the answer right now. I can either go away and find out the answer, or we could do some research to figure it out together, what do you think?"*

Fill their cups!

We all have needs that have to be met each day, or in another term, cups that need to be filled each day, and when our cups are full, we are more resilient and capable of dealing with change and distress. We have cups to fill, such as hunger, thirst, sleep, emotional connection, safety, attention etc. When we are able to fill our children's cups (and our own), stress levels are reduced, so by ensuring that your child's cup is filled each day they will feel less overwhelmed and are better able to manage changes. Or alternatively before you notify them about an upcoming change, you might check first that all their cups have been filled. This could be really practical stuff like making sure they aren't hungry, sleepy or feeling unwell.

Gratitude

When we intentionally focus on the positives in our life it changes the way we see and process things in our world. Gratitude doesn't even have to be about the big stuff, it could be about small things we notice each day, like helping your child to notice fresh smelling sheets on their bed, that you made their favorite dinner, that their brother/sister shared a toy with them, that they coloured in the lines or got over 70% on a math test. So, if you bring in a daily gratitude challenge into your family's life, you are not only giving your child the skills to see the positives intentionally but the act of being grateful improves mental wellbeing and resilience, which in turn increases resilience and our capacity to weather the storms.

There are lots of ways that you can support your child to cope with big changes in their life, but the biggest take away is that we can't protect them entirely from change. We as parents and caregivers need to help our children develop the skills to cope with and make it through tough times that are a part of life.

Change is tough on children, and adults too. So ensure that you are also looking after yourself during challenging times, because not only will you be able to better cope and sit with your child's big emotions that will invariably appear, but also your child will see you looking after yourself and they will learn that self-care is important and understand that they too can prioritize and look after themselves when things are overwhelming and rough.

STARTING SCHOOL OR DAYCARE

Transitioning kids into childcare/day-care or school marks the start of a new adventure! It's a whole new environment for our kids to navigate with different toys, unknown kids and carers, plus different routines. It's hard for parents also as we have to take a huge leap of faith and learn to trust someone else to care for our kids (cue Mom-guilt!).

Some children will adjust pretty quickly to their new setting. Perhaps your little one is very social and loves the interaction with other children and carers/educators, or maybe they are quite relaxed, independent, and don't mind taking on the challenge. However, many children can be uncertain, worried, or scared. It's not uncommon to see children clinging to their parents at drop-off, which absolutely pulls at the heartstrings. But here's what you don't see: Most of the time, just a few minutes after you leave, they have joined their group or class and have become happily distracted by something else. It's the process of separating and saying goodbye that triggers the distress.

Transition into Childcare

Separation anxiety as your child transitions into childcare is really common given their development. Research suggests that separation anxiety increases until a child is about 15 months of age and peaks at around 18 months. This is why sometimes your child may have been attending childcare quite happily and then all of a sudden, separation anxiety starts! Rest assured that this is just a sign that your little one has reached a developmental milestone and is now more aware that you are leaving, and that you still exist even when you are not in sight. Thankfully, somewhere between 18-24 months, their expressive and receptive language skills begin to rapidly develop, which helps them to better understand that their parents will come back later, and allows them to communicate more effectively with others. As a result, this is typically when we see our kids forming stronger friendships with peers and relationships with their educators.

<u>Preparing younger children for childcare</u>

The more we do to prepare our kids for childcare, the better! That's why it's really common for many childcare centers to have an orientation process. This typically involves parents and kids spending a few hours together at the center, which is usually repeated 2-3 times. Together you can explore the rooms, play with other children, spend time with the educators, and get familiar with the environment. It's really important that when you do orientation, you put any of your own worries aside and show your children that you trust the educators, that it's a safe place to be, and you're happy to be there. If you show uncertainty, kids will often interpret this as childcare being a negative place, which would understandably create feelings of anxiety.

Once orientation is complete, your little one should be familiar with the childcare center and have a few positive associations. If your little one is still quite ambivalent about attending, even with you, you may need a few more orientation sessions. But if they seem comfortable, your child is ready to attend on their own. From this point onwards, it's helpful to forewarn your kids about the days they are going to childcare – don't spring it on them! In the morning tell them they're going to childcare and remind them of the fun things they may do with their friends and carers e.g. *"Today you get to see Willian and Lily at childcare! Remember how you played in the sandpit with them the other day? That was so fun!"*

If it helps, have a few photos on the fridge as a reminder.

Tips for Childcare Drop-Off

Once you're at the gates or front door, be sure to have your child greeted by someone they are familiar with. If having a particular toy helps them, or a security blanket (comforter), that's fine! Keep your farewells brief, the more you linger, the longer they have to worry and get worked up. It's easier for your little one if you give a quick farewell, and let them get on with the fun. Most of the time, once the parent leaves, even if they cry initially, they can be quickly redirected and will be smiling again and playing within a few minutes. If your child remains distressed, childcare will likely call you (you can request this) and you can have a few more orientation sessions.

School Transition

For older children, the process of transitioning into school can be slightly different than those moving into childcare. Kids who have never been to childcare or kindergarten may be more uncertain, which is common and understandable, but this isn't always the case. Many kids have learned about school and are quite excited to start a new adventure!

Common reasons for school anxiety and (potential) refusal

Most of us try to avoid things which make us feel uncomfortable, and kids do the same! If they are uncertain, scared, or nervous about school, there may be some resistance to attending. If their resistance to attending school occurs before they commence, most of the time it's because they aren't sure what to expect or what a day will be like. They may be wondering who their teacher will be, who the other children are, worry about making new friends, or how to navigate the physical school grounds. If your child has been attending school happily and then there is a change in their behavior, chances are something has happened which is causing worry. Perhaps they have had a negative encounter with another child, the teacher disciplined them and they feel bad, or maybe they are starting to compare themselves to others and are worried about their performance at school. I don't know anyone who has survived school without experiencing a degree of self-consciousness at some point.

<u>How to prepare kids for school transition</u>

Most children, before starting at a primary school, will attend at least one orientation day. This is their opportunity to meet their teachers and spend a few hours exploring the school with their soon-to-be classmates. If your child attended childcare in the same locality as the school, there is a good chance they may already know a couple of other children, which can be comforting. After any orientation day, be sure to speak with your child about all the amazing things they saw and what they are looking forward to. If you have the ability to access any photos of the school, print these off and talk about them, and keep them somewhere visible. Talk about any friends they made, and store this in your memory for when the school term starts. To help build familiarity with the school, if possible, visit over the holidays. Play on the school equipment or shoot some hoops on the basketball courts. Let them take you on a school tour!

It's also important to talk about what to expect from a day at school. Speak about school assembly, how there is a bell that sounds to indicate when it's time to play at recess and lunchtime, and how there are different rooms for different classes, such as a music room or the library.

If your child raises any concerns, pause and listen. If you don't really understand why they are worried, ask more questions! If we give a solution too quickly, it's often dismissed because we haven't listened and it's not helpful. So take the time to listen, understand, and validate (e.g. *"Ahh, I see, you're worried that people won't be your friend because you're a little bit shy"*). Then provide some reassurance and start the problem-solving process (e.g. *"You know, being shy also means you're a very good listener, which is very important! Maybe we can practice how you can say hi to new friends in class?")*

Tip for School Drop Off

As much as children will complain about many of their routines, they actually provide a sense of comfort because it keeps things predictable. On a school day, ensure you keep your kids' mornings as routine as possible. Wake at a certain time, get dressed, breakfast, bags packed, and off to school at a certain time. Whether you walk or drive to school, ensure the journey is a positive one. Talk about what's on for the day, for both of you, and what you plan to do after school. For instance, you could say something like *"You have music and sports today, that'll be fun! I'm working today too. After work I'll come and pick you up, and then we'll head home and we can organize pasta for dinner, how does that sound?"* If possible, drop your child off at the same area every day. If they have a good friend already, see if they can meet your child at the same drop-off area. For children with very heightened separation anxiety, many parents find it helpful to walk their children into the school office or classroom, and hand them over to a teacher they trust. Alternatively, sometimes the school staff can distract your kids by giving them a task to complete, such as putting paper in the photocopy machine or running an errand, which can take their mind off saying goodbye, give them a sense of accomplishment, and ease them into the school environment.

If Your Child Continues to Experience Anxiety

There could be something more going on if anxiety persists for more than a few weeks. Perhaps they have had a negative experience that needs to be discussed and worked through, or maybe there is someone or something they are afraid of. For younger children, this complicates things as they will often not have the verbal skills to tell you what is upsetting them. If you find yourself in this situation, it can be helpful to ask childcare workers to keep a logbook of when your child becomes upset and what's happening at the time. If you want to engage a healthcare practitioner, such as a child psychologist, they may be able to go to childcare and complete observations to help you identify the stressor and provide you, and the educators, with additional strategies to help your little one overcome their fears.

If your child is attending school, try having some time together to talk about their fears. Even though their worries may seem trivial or silly to us, we need to keep in mind that it's very serious and real for them. They haven't had years of life experience and the opportunity to develop coping skills like we have. Find a time when you are both free and can speak uninterrupted. Sometimes doing an activity together can help facilitate conversation. Ask your child about what they like about school – an icebreaker. When you're ready to bring up their difficulties, try starting the conversation by normalizing and relating to their distress. For example, "*When I was your age, I had some trouble getting used to going to school too. It was such a big place and I felt a bit lost. It took me a few weeks to feel confident in going. Do you ever feel like that?*"

As your child opens up, be curious. Ask questions in a gentle, soft voice, nod your head to show you understand. Don't try to offer solutions until you have a firm understanding of their worries. Once you have collected all the information you need, ask your child how they feel and if they have thought of any solutions. If they have a good solution, you can help them finetune it or implement it. For instance, if they think meeting their best friend at the gate would be helpful, you can help to organize this by chatting with their friends' parents, or the school teacher, who could help organize this. If your child doesn't have any ideas, ask them if they want to brainstorm with you and problem solve together. Creating a plan together is likely to be more helpful and empowering to your children than if you simply take over the situation. Again, if you feel that you can't get to the bottom of things, enlist the help of a professional. Many schools will have on-site counselors, welfare workers, chaplains or psychologists on standby to help you!

If your child's school doesn't have access to support, have a chat with your doctor and discuss other referral options.

SECTION 3

Development

BEHAVIORAL AND DEVELOPMENTAL LEAPS BETWEEN THE AGES OF 3 AND 6 – FOSTERING STRONG RELATIONSHIPS

It's important to understand that although these are key markers or guidelines for development not every child will develop at the same speed. However, they are typical behaviors or changes we notice, so if your child is not meeting these guides or displaying most of the behaviors we would expect to see, it is important to consult your GP or trusted health professional.

We will look at four key areas of development; Physical, Cognitive, Language and Social/Emotional as well as how you can support your child through each stage and age, whilst building strong relationships.

It might seem automatic that when your child is born you will experience a reciprocal and strong relationship, but that isn't always true. We need to build a relationship with our child just like any other person. Relationship-building refers to the establishment of emotional connections with other people. This process commences at birth, and early relationships are based on trust and intimacy. In the early days and months, it's very simple; our children cry and we respond. This teaches them that not only can they trust that someone (you) will help meet their needs, but that their distress is something that is manageable.

Through consistent and safe relationships, children discover who they are as individuals and also learn about other's needs. It is essential that early relationships with children focus on meeting their emotional, physical and cognitive needs and when our little people have a lived experience where people strive to understand them and enjoy their present they can see and explore their world with enthusiasm and curiosity. This is why it's important to understand the developmental stages our children are going through so that we can meet them where they are at and provide opportunities to not only help them develop but also, simultaneously build a loving, safe and respectful relationship with them.

KEY DEVELOPMENTAL MILESTONES: AGE 3 – 4 YEARS

Physical Milestones – at this stage our children are working hard to finesse and refine their motor skills. We typically see more pronounced development of their gross motor skills at this age, but they will start demonstrating some fine motor skills also (small movements of their muscles).

Gross Motor Skills

- Hopping
- Jumping
- Balancing on one foot
- Running (less tripping over their own feet)
- Step up/down stairs using one foot after the other
- May be able to catch a large ball (most of the time)
- Pedal a bike/trike
- Climb

Fine Motor Skills

- Drawing a line
- Drawing a circle
- Turning the pages of a book one at a time
- Open doors, twist handles or lids
- Using mixed media (pens, crayons, markers)
- Be able to manipulate toys with small moving parts (buttons, levers, wheels)

- Build towers or construct things using blocks (balancing or fitting them with other blockers) – around 6+ blocks

Supporting Physical Milestones

- Improve your child's balance by putting tape on the floor in a shape for them to follow (stepping on the tape in a straight line).
- Put out hula hoops on the floor (lying flat on the ground) and have them jump from one hoop to the next – aiming to jump into the middle of the hoop.
- Take them on a mindfulness walk outside
- Let your child have time to free play outside without shoes and socks if possible. We want our kids to have the experience of walking barefoot to improve their balance and to help them respond to different feelings under their feet. This improves their gross motor skills and muscle tone if they walk over different types of ground (rocky, steps, grass, slopes etc).
- Practice coordination by engaging two handed tasks – rolling dough into a snake (using two hands to work together to push and roll the dough).
- Lay out puzzles for them to find and play with
- Play dress ups. Not only are dress ups great to engage imagination, but they also give sneaky opportunities to practice fine motor skills required for dressing themselves (pick dress ups with ties, buttons, zips etc). It becomes a game not a chore to learn about caring for themselves.
- Threading or playing with beads – improves hand eye coordination required to thread beads onto string (this is an activity to be closely supervised)
- Finger feeding – putting a variety of foods that can be finger fed on a plate is important. Not only do our kids learn to feed themselves but they are practicing the pincer grasp (thumb and first finger pinching together) which is a precursor skill required for holding a pen and

writing.

Cognitive Milestones – at the age of three our children are starting to understand their world in new ways and are learning how to group or link objects/things in their environment. They also start learning to problem solve and tackle problems creatively.

- Name primary colors (red, green, blue) and most other colors in the rainbow
- Be able to count up to at least 10
- Start counting small groups of things (being able to recite numbers in order is different than being able to identify how many of an object is present)
- Start understanding timeframes – like morning, night etc. And may understand or recognise days of the week
- Start being able to compare things - things being different or the same (mentally grouping, sorting and linking objects and people in their environment)
- Follow three step directions (simple direction) like grab your spoon, sit at the table and start eating your breakfast.
- Ask "why?" ...a lot! Your child's curiosity is developing and they are interested in how their world works.

<u>Supporting Cognitive Milestones</u>

- Cook together and ask for their help – you can make learning to count fun and turn reciting numbers into a practical application. Count together (aloud) how many cups or spoons you need of something as you make a recipe together.
- Read your child lots of books and also ask them to try and tell you what they think is happening based on the picture on the page. This capacity to interpret information and make sense of it develops their cognitive skills (as they use current knowledge to help them make sense of what they can see).

- Play memory games where your child has to recall what or where an object is. One example might be a memory card game where pairs of cards are shuffled and turned over (a blank side of card is facing upwards) and you take turns to flip the cards and try to match pairs. You could also put some objects on a table (dice, a feather, a small ball, a figurine etc) and get them to take a good look at the items and recite them back to you. Once they have seen what's on the table, get them to turn around whilst you remove an item (don't let them see which one you have removed) and then ask them to name which item you removed.
- Draw up or find a calendar to pop on the fridge. A month-long calendar as well as a daily schedule are two different ways to help them learn. You can use both the monthly calendar and the daily schedule to track important things which are meaningful for your child. For example – write kindy/school days or day care day on the calendar and tell them which days they attend. Pop in sports or other activities like parties etc and they can count down to the exciting event by tracking which day it is, and how many days are left until the day arrives. A daily schedule can help your child make sense of morning, noon and night by adding in key elements of their daily routine and helping them to understand which time of day equates to which activity. For example; in the morning we brush our teeth and get dressed and eat breakfast. In the evening we eat dinner, read a story, have a bath and go to bed.

Language Milestones – your child's receptive and expressive language is starting to boom at this age. Receptive language refers to how much they receive or understand in communication, and expressive language refers to how they use language to express themselves and communicate. It is the norm for our younger kids to be much better at understanding a wide range of words than being able to accurately use them yet.

- By three years most children will be able to use 5-6-word sentences and two or three sentence conversations
- People will be able to understand most of what they say
- They will still gesture (pointing etc) to try and get their point across
- Grammar is usually correct, but they might still struggle with exceptions to the rule. For example; one orange or three oranges will usually be correct, but they may yet know that its mice, not mouses (which is an exception to the rule of multiples)
- They will ask lots of "w" questions (who, what, when, where, why) as they are curious about the world around them
- They know their name, and the names of close family and friends
- They can name most of the everyday things/objects around them

<u>Supporting language milestones</u>

- Narrate! It might feel a little silly, but as you go about your day narrate your actions and thoughts. "I'm going over to the sink to put my cup away". Our kids are always listening and copying what we say and do, so when we narrate our actions, we are giving a lesson without having to sit them down and teach them what is a sink and what is a cup.
- Use lots of descriptions when you talk about objects. "Can you pass me that red, stripy t-shirt?"
- Read them lots of stories. As other people use language in different ways, reading stories exposes them to a variety of speech patterns and new words.
- Encourage them to play dress ups or role play. When they take on another character, they also modify their language to align with what they think the other person might sound like (or how they express themselves). It

can give them an opportunity to play with language and practice expressing their thoughts in a different way.

Social and Emotional Milestones

- Our children are going through a huge rate of development in relation to their emotions.
- They will be able to start expressing and learning to identify their emotions using simple words (good, bad, mad, sad, happy etc)
- Some three-year old's may also be able to identify emotions in others and may start to show empathy or concern for others' emotional state.
- They move from parallel play (side by side but not engaged) to cooperative play (playing with another and working towards a common goal or aim)
- Our kids may be overtly interested in theirs or others' genitals (this is a normal stage of development). See below for safe and appropriate ways of supporting them to understand and learn about their bodies.
- They will be interested in new things but are learning to be more discerning and might be hesitant to try new things
- Turn taking is progressing! They may not like taking turns (who does?) but they are learning that this is an expectation in life to share and give others a turn.
- Role play! Our children are starting to play pretend and in particular are trying out new and different characters.
- Independence is huge at this age and this desire to "do it myself" can result in power struggles. It's a tricky stage of development because our kids might want to be independent but they might not be able to safely act/ behave independently yet.

<u>Supporting Social and Emotional Milestones</u>

- Give your child as many (safe) opportunities as you can to let them make choices and be independent, in particular activities where they are looking after themselves. Set out a few options of breakfast cereal, ask them what movie they would like to watch as a family, give them a choice of puzzles to play with. One situation that gives many parents a challenge is self-dressing. You might struggle with your child selecting their clothes as they don't pick weather or situation appropriate clothes...so fill separate drawers or shelves with clothes for certain occasions (warm clothes in one drawer, summer clothes in another etc). This way they can only choose from appropriate clothes you have already vetted, but more importantly they will have the experience of being independent and making their own decisions.

- It's my body! Your child is naturally interested in their bodies and self-discovery. It can be tricky to find a good balance between being open about our bodies and also ensuring that they understand that it's their body, and that certain body parts are private. This is also the age to teach our children about consent. Sounds like these are quite big terms for little children, but we can use language and discuss things in terms they will understand.
    - Always use the anatomical words, penis and vagina. If your child uses the right words and is comfortable using them it lessens the idea that our genitals or bodies are something to be ashamed of (which they aren't!!).
    - Teach them that body parts under their clothes are private and no-one else should touch them except themselves...nor should they touch anyone else's. It is also important to send the message that it's their body and no-one else can touch any of their body parts (covered in clothes or not) without their permission. And this is where we come to consent.
    - Don't force your child to hug, kiss, high five, hold hands or touch anybody else if they don't want

to. You can invite them to make a choice "We are going to say goodbye to grandma now, how would you like to say goodbye? A hug? A kiss? You choose." This is the early stages of teaching consent, inviting them to make a choice about physical contact and respecting their decision. This helps them understand important boundaries about their bodies and other peoples.

- Name your own emotions as you experience them, as well as how you cope. Our kids are sponges and they are always picking up on our actions and behaviors....and copying them. Tell them how you are feeling, why and what you are going to do next to help you manage "I'm feeling really frustrated right now because I spilled the pot of dinner. Because I'm feeling a bit angry, I'm going to take a few deep breaths before I go and start cleaning up." It's important to give our children the names for their emotions, because when they understand the confusing sensations in their bodies (as different emotions) they feel less confused and feel more in control and better able to cope. This means less tantrums because our little ones don't feel as overwhelmed by their feelings. Winning!!

BUILDING A STRONG RELATIONSHIP WITH YOUR 3-4 YEAR OLD

Ever heard of the term "Three-nager?". The term was coined because we are out of the "Terrible Twos" (phew), but we are entering the next stage of development where our children are growing bigger, they have more vocabulary and are learning new things every day...but they are still little and get easily overwhelmed. It's also a stage of development where we might be seeing a battle of the wills. Our little people are desperate to be independent, but they aren't always equipped physically or emotionally to make the best choices for themselves.

To build a strong relationship with your three-year-old it is really about consistent boundaries, picking your battles and giving them lots of opportunities to be (safely) independent. Many parents either want to put in lots of boundaries and rules (in hopes of taming their toddlers) or struggle with the frequent challenges for power. I don't say this in a negative way, it's very normal and appropriate for our children to rally against rules and boundaries. They are learning about consistency, what they can get away with and expectations that differ based on the person or situation...this is all part of figuring out the rules of the world they live in. It's also very normal that parents are challenged and frustrated by the behavior of their 3-4-year-old children.

Boundaries, boundaries, boundaries! It is essential that we give our children clear and consistent boundaries, not just because it gives them clarity about what is appropriate or not, which helps their social development and adjustment but it also helps our children feel safe and secure. When we are consistent about rules and boundaries our children know what to expect from us, and conversely what we or a situation requires of them and this clarity helps them to feel secure. It's easy to be inconsistent, and it happens to the best of us, so don't judge yourself too harshly, but absolutely make it your best intention to be firm with your boundaries/expectations. If your child feels secure, they are also less likely to become distressed and overwhelmed (tantrums!) in new situations, when a rule is being applied or if you put a boundary in place.

It is also tempting to go the other way and become too caught up on the rules. But having too many rules is confusing for our kids because it takes many (many) instances for new information to sink in. Generally, it's best to have some bigger or overarching rules and try to avoid sweating the small stuff. Your big stuff will usually be aligned with your values and morals; treating others respectfully, being honest etc. So definitely ensure those expectations are being firmly reinforced; however, the little daily skirmishes can be minimized. So, your child wants to wear their tiara to the shops, they want to mix all the separate coloured playdough together into one big brown blob, or refuse to brush their hair one morning. Ok, these might be outside of your own comfort zone, but in essence do they really truly matter. Pick your battles parents!

KEY DEVELOPMENTAL MILESTONES: 4 – 5 YEARS

Physical Milestones – at this stage our children are starting to become more coordinated because their eyesight is continuing to improve, as is their muscle tone and control over big muscle groups. They are also building on their pincer grasp and getting better with fine details or manipulating small objects.

Gross Motor Skills

- Turn door handles
- Instead of just being able to run in a line they are starting to bring in other muscle groups and can stop, start, jump, turn etc whilst running
- Use a ladder
- Jump with two feet
- Throw, bounce and catch a ball
- Start being able to steer and pedal a tricycle or bike

Fine Motor Skills

- Draw shapes that may be good representations of letters; some might be exact copies, and others might be distinct marks that bare a good resemblance to letters
- They will start moving the pen/pencil on a page in the shape of "M"s or mountains to represent "writing"
- Starting to be able to manipulate scissors in an intentional way

- They can start to cross the midline
    - The midline of the body is an invisible line down the middle of the body separating the left and right sides. Being able to cross the midline means that they can reach across the middle of their body with either their arms or legs to complete an activity/ task on the other side of the body (i.e. using their dominant hand let's say their right hand to reach diagonally across their body to pick up a puzzle piece on their left hand side, being able to sit cross legged on the floor, etc)
- Get dressed with little help and can handle zippers, Velcro, or clips, although laces and buttons are likely to still evade them

<u>Supporting Physical Milestones</u>

- Give your child heaps of opportunities for messy play like playing with arts and crafts, mud kitchens, slime etc! Playing with lots of different materials whilst crafting, or giving them lots of textures to play with will help them develop their sensory skills. For example; knowing how to gently pick up small beads requires a different physical skill than squeezing playdough between their hands. Not only do they learn how to process different textures and respond accordingly but it's also a lot of fun, and kids don't realize they are learning.
- Set up puzzles or games (like clapping games) that requires them to reach across their midline
- When you take them to the playground, instead of just running around, encourage them to climb. Climbing ladders or ropes or up climbing walls requires our children to coordinate all of their limbs and strengthens their core. This helps them with other gross motor activities and general strength and coordination.
- Support them to get dressed themselves. Try not to rush in if they struggle with their buttons or zips, let

them try first and encourage them to take increasing responsibility for getting themselves ready for the day or ready for bed.

Cognitive Milestones – between the ages of 4 and 5 our children start to consider the world outside of their own little bubble. Whereas previously children wouldn't necessarily be aware of things they can't directly see, they can now start to apply their understanding and knowledge to the wider world. They are particularly interested in relationships and sorting, comparing and contrasting things to more fully understand how things fit or work together.

- You might notice your child can sort things by simple attributes such as color, shape or size and can order them (smallest to biggest etc)
- They also start comparing things – notable gender or size
- Understanding logic and consequences. This process doesn't truly complete until our early 20s (when the prefrontal cortex of the brain responsible for logical decision-making puts on its finishing touches) but our children are starting to identify that actions have consequences.
- Children of this age can understand ideas like later, soon, tomorrow, more, less
- They are starting to move from being able to recite numbers up to 20 to being able to count things/objects in a group (i.e. "I can see five biscuits")
- Start recognising objects in pictures on TV or photos that exist in real life. This can be confusing as they are also starting to learn about reality and fantasy and may still struggle with ideas of make-believe stories or tv shows about monsters, witches, etc. However, they are becoming more concrete in their understanding which is reality and which is made up.
- Their attention span is increasingly and they may be able to stick to an activity for 10 or more minutes

Supporting Cognitive Milestones

- Board games! Pull out the simple dice games. Your child will be able to start counting the dots on a dice piece and will be able to grasp moving the required number of spaces.
- Card games like UNO or snap are great games to play. They can start matching colors or shapes to create required "pairs"
- Delayed gratification – learning to wait and be patient is an important skill for our children to learn. Set up a project you both do that doesn't result in an immediate gain like planting seeds or doing some baking. There are lots of steps in between and then a fair bit of waiting between the start of these activities and the "reward". You are helping them to learn to stay focussed, and take immediate steps/action for some later reward. Being able to delay gratification is shown in later years to improve our children's educational attainment and financial stability (being able to save or having healthy spending habits) amongst other things.
- Consequences. Ensure that you ask your child for their opinion on what a logical consequence might be when reading stories or watching a tv show. Ask them "What do you think is going to happen next?" when you reach a crisis point in the story you are following. We want our kids to start thinking about consequences which helps them with decision making.
- Play "guess what" games – think about an object and get your child to guess what you are imagining. Start describing it to your child in the most abstract sense, getting more specific with each description. This requires them to not only hold several pieces of information in their brain, but they also need to access their knowledge about topics or groupings to try and figure out what you are imagining. For example; I'm an

animal, I have 4 legs, I have fur, I like to eat fish, I say meow. What am I?

Language Milestones – language is really exploding at this age. Their capacity to use and understand language is starting to even out, whereas previously they understood more than they could verbally communicate or express. They are also starting to be able to manipulate language; rhyming, using humor, combining multiple thoughts or ideas in their sentences and communications.

- Around the age of four children will be able to speak in sentences of up to 5 or 6 words but by the time they reach closer to five years, their sentences are more complex and they can say around 9 words.
- Your child will start to enjoy using language and will make up songs, jokes, rhyme, tell made up stories or tell you what they are thinking
- They can follow instructions of usually 2 -3 steps like "Can you please grab me your shoes, your socks and bring them here so I can help you put them on."
- Other people will generally understand most of the words they say, but they may struggle with the sounds; "s", "w" and "r".

Supporting language milestones

- Correct by modeling. If your child is using an incorrect word, or is struggling with their pronunciation it's important to address it. Beyond the age of 5 speech issues can start to impact their literacy and also intelligibility (can other people understand what they are trying to say). When they have trouble expressing themselves it can cause frustration, nervousness around communicating, literacy issues and even loss of confidence. Instead of drawing their attention to the correct way of saying something, just repeat it back to them in the correct way. For example, if they say "Can you pass me the wed [red] car?" you might respond "Yes I can pass you the red car" making sure to emphasize the correct sound of the "r".

- Create fun games with rhyming, trying to make up silly stories or if you aren't sure, read a rhyming picture book to them.
- When you speak with your child try to carve out some uninterrupted time and ask them all about their favorite topics or interest areas. Make sure that you are really looking at them and they have a chance to see your face when you are speaking. Being able to visibly see other people make sounds and hear how others use language is one of the best ways to improve communication.

Social and Emotional Milestones – this age is all about personality! Your little person is really starting to come into their own, they are starting the transition to school and socially there are big adjustments where the core family cease to be the only relationship groups they are in; social relationships definitely start to take on increased importance. Children of this age are also starting to learn how to cooperate and work collaboratively because of their new interest and investment in friendships.

- We might start to see less tantrums as our children are more capable of demonstrating and expressing a wider range of emotions. They are also likely to have increased language to tell you why they feel a certain way which reduces their frustration, and in turn reduces the likelihood of tantrums. However, with this being said, tantrums will still exist and changes to routines or lack of control over a situation may be particularly triggering.
- Social interest increased as this age, our children want to start expanding their relationships and start placing more importance on friendships.
- Because of an increased desire to be social and make friends, our children are also learning how to cooperate and negotiate. This is because they start to understand

that to make friends and build relationships it is a two-way street of reciprocity.

- Lies are a normal part of child development. Before the age of four, children are still learning how to differentiate between reality and fantasy, or their intense emotional reactions can result in big/dramatic (and possibly untrue statements), so they aren't truly telling lies. However, from four onwards we start to see increased language (to express themselves more articulately), desire to be seen as good and avoid trouble which can culminate in intentional telling of lies.
- Children at this age start to become more aware of their gender and generally start to associate with peers of a particular gender or show a gender role preference.

<u>Supporting Social and Emotional Milestones</u>

- Giving children an opportunity to learn how to turn-take is essential at this age. We are all naturally egocentric and don't necessarily want to share; however, as our kids enter school and desire to build strong and positive relationships, they do need to learn that not everything can go their way, or they might have to share and take turns. One great way to practice these skills can be:
    - Using an object to represent whose turn it is to speak. For example; you might use a toy microphone or a teddy. Whoever is holding the teddy gets to speak without interruption, and there is a time limit (set the limit based on your child's attention span) before they either have to put the toy down or pass it along for someone else to speak. We encourage our children to be patient and take turns in conversations. We also can also use the opportunity to model what actively listening looks and feels like which builds their social capacity.
    - Choose one night of the week to have a family night. Each person in the family takes turns

choosing an event, food, music etc for the evening for the rest of the family to enjoy. Not only will your child learn about turn taking, but they will also start to build on their empathy when they consider different options when it's their turn and whether their family will enjoy their choices.

- If your child is telling lies, try to avoid shaming them, this might exacerbate lies in the future as they can become secretive and further wanting to avoid getting in trouble (increasing their lies). Instead you might gently question further or even address the behavior behind the lie "That seems interesting to me, can you tell me how that happened?", "Hmmm, I'm not sure that your sister did hit you, can you try and explain to me again what happened?", "I can see that you really don't want to get in trouble, and so you have told me that the cat knocked over my favorite vase. Does that sound right?" After the initial heat of the moment has passed, we need to speak to our kids about the importance of honesty and why we shouldn't lie.
- Play the feelings in my body activity
- Narrate and model your own feelings, reactions to situations as well as your coping strategies. "I feel really frustrated that I dropped the milk and now I have to clean it up. I think I'll take three deep breaths and then when I feel calm again, I'll come and clean it up." This externalization of your own internal experiences gives them examples and reference points for their own internal experiences. When they can make sense of their emotions, they are less likely to become overwhelmed by them.

BUILDING A STRONG RELATIONSHIP WITH YOUR 4-5 YEAR OLD

Relationship building is key at this age, not only between you and your child, but also their relationships with other people outside of your immediate circle. To build a strong relationship with your four – five-year-old it's important to spend some quality time with them, it doesn't have to be hours and hours, but the quality of the interaction really matters. Make sure to lock some uninterrupted time into your schedule, if it's possible to have the same time each week or day your child will enjoy the predictability. Be fully present and allow for unstructured time together, where you don't have any other purpose than being with them and enjoying their company.

They are developing their personalities and unique interests, so spend this time finding all about who they are becoming as a unique individual. Ask them about their favorite books, tv shows, games, animals etc and see where the conversation goes. And then listen, and I mean really listen, with your whole body. Turn to face them, make eye contact, soften your body posture, get down on their level and ask questions that show you heard what they said. When you really take the time to listen to your child you are showing them how much you value them and that what they have to say is important. If they learn to trust that you are genuinely interested in what they have to say they are more likely to take this trust right through to adolescence and confide in you about the big stuff you are really going to want to be aware of. So, listen in now, to build the trust for later.

Boundaries are key at this age. You want to encourage independence (incrementally and age appropriate of course) but you also need to set some clear rules. It can be a tricky balance to get right, too many rules and children can lose self-esteem as they don't feel capable or trusted, and not enough rules and children feel scared and often end up trying to control situations if they don't feel the adult in their life is putting in enough containment or safety. It is essential to have a few key rules or expectations that underpin your family values, things like honesty, respect, kindness etc. as well as a few specific rules around safety and communication, things like; you must always hold a grownup's hand to cross the road etc. But parents…pick your battles! With a four-year-old you could be battling the little things all day, every day if you aren't careful, and this will erode your strong relationship. So, decide in advance with anyone else who shares key caregiving responsibilities of your child what the non-negotiables are so that you can all be consistent. And then try not to sweat the small stuff, your child is becoming increasingly independent and wanting to feel a sense of control over their world, which in turn improves their sense of self-esteem because they feel capable. So as long as their choices don't interfere or cross your non-negotiables, is there any harm in letting them wear a tiara to the shops, eat their cereal without milk, brush their teeth after they get into their pajamas instead of beforehand? Probably not, so let some of the small things slide and save your energy for the big/important things.

KEY DEVELOPMENTAL MILESTONES: 5 – 6 YEARS

Physical Milestones – you will notice your child making big physical gains, being more coordinated and skilful in their movements. This is also the age where we start to see hand dominance for key tasks and they will be more accurate and independent when completing their daily living tasks.

Gross Motor Skills

- Use their bodies and all four limbs separately but also in more coordinated ways by combining gross motor skills - like swimming, dancing, skipping rope, playing netball or baseball etc.
- They will start testing their limitations of their bodies – doing cartwheels, forward rolls, jumping from heights and in general being more daring.
- They can usually walk one foot directly in front of the other, on a balance beam or in a line.
- Balance on one foot and start to hop

Fine Motor Skills

- Pencil grip has been perfected (or nearly perfect) in a tripod position with two fingers and a thumb on the pencil
- Scissor use is improved and they may be able to cut a straight line or a basic shape

- They will favor one hand over the other for most tasks and will use their key hand with more dexterity
- Cutlery use is more precise – they will be able to cut their own food and scoop up small objects (like peas). Although imperfect, they will be able to do it independent
- Activities like dressing, including tying laces, doing buttons and also being able to do things like wiping and washing after going to the toilet.

<u>Supporting Physical Milestones</u>

- Play music – whether it be playing musical instruments (which requires memory of keys or patterns and engages fine motor skills) or whether it be dancing to music (coordination, steps or rhythms to follow) children will gain lots of skills from playing music.
- Make playdough and play games with it! Yes, it can be fun for children to mold playdough into objects, but they are also strengthening their hands muscles which is important for fine motor skills like writing. You can play games which help with other types of development, for example roll a dice and ask your child to count the numbers on the dice and then make the correct number of playdough balls to coincide, for example if they roll a 5, then they would make 5 balls. You could also play a guessing game with dough, write down some animals or everyday objects on a piece of paper and pop them into a hat. Take turns picking out of the hat and making whatever item you selected using playdough, add a time for a bit of a competitive edge
- Play outside! Being outside means your child will be exposed to lots of different surfaces. Their bodies need to respond to uneven terrain by clenching or flexing different muscles to keep them balanced. As they adjust to the different ground, they will improve their core strength as well as general muscle tone and balance.

Cognitive Milestones – children will be able to start thinking creatively and will be starting to grasp some early academic concepts like reading short words, counting, understanding the alphabet and sounds of letters.

- They will be able to categorize objects with more finesse than at age four, being able to name and sort things by size, shape, color
- Recite up to the number 20 and be able to count groups of up to 10 objects
- Reading orientation – be able to visually identify what way up a book goes, from looking at the text, and also being able to understand that in English we read left to right and from top to the bottom of the page. If a language other than English is spoken or read at home, this applies to whichever direction reading goes.
- They can understand that stories have a beginning, middle/conflict and end and will start telling their own made up stories.
- Thinking through and planning activities will be better executed. They will know what objects are required for their activity and will consider what steps they need to undertake to complete their project.
- Their attention span has increased and they may be able to stick to a single activity for longer than 15 minutes
- Increased capacity to understand cause and effect.

Supporting Cognitive Milestones

- Set up activities to get them counting, sorting and learning about relationships objects have with one another. Get them to sort their pencils into coloured groups (all the blues together, all the greens etc), ask them to count all the red cars you see on a drive together, get them to sort their toys from smallest to largest.
- Print some pictures of simple stories like the three bears and goldilocks and tell them the story. See if they can

match the storyline in order based on the pictures that represent the story.

- Create pictorial lists to help them with their planning skills. For example; print out some pictures of daily living tasks and laminate them, you can then blu tack them to the fridge in order of their getting ready routine, or create a board with sticky Velcro dots that they can use to create an order/routine for their day. They can then refer to the list/order to help them get ready independently. Having a list, they can refer to can also stop arguments or constant parental reminders to move onto the next step in getting ready.

Language Milestones – five to six-year-old children are talking very quickly and have an extensive vocabulary that they aren't afraid to use. Children at this age like to talk about anything and everything...and they like talking! They will start to be able to use their language to such a degree that they can pose arguments to substantiate their opinions.

- "Because" – our children love to use this word to structure their arguments and opinions and when they try to reason with others. They might not yet have the capacity to get more specific than "because" as a backup to their argument.
- They can use plurals and pronouns correctly.
- Comparisons and opposites. Our children can start to use their language to explore comparisons. *"That coloured marble is bigger than that other marble."*
- Children of this age can understand and use thousands of words.
- Following instructions is improving. They can follow simple multi-step requests or activities.

<u>Supporting language milestones</u>

- Play opposites games – there are lots of games on the market you can purchase, but you can also go online and print out images of opposite pairs, like; big versus small, tall versus short, messy versus clean, in versus out (or on), empty versus full. The list goes on. Ask them to match pairs of opposites, but don't leave it there, extend the game and ask them how they know that was the answer and to describe why they are different. Not only are you helping them learn about groupings/ relationships/comparison, you are also improving their capacity to express their thoughts and put forward rational arguments to support their ideas.

- Play eye spy! If your child is not recognising letters yet you can use colors or descriptions to structure your game of Eye Spy.
- Focus on phonics and also sound word games. Phonological awareness refers to the sounds (phonemes) in words, for example dog, is three distinct sounds d-o-g, and we sound it out the way we pronounce it, not the way we say the alphabet (dee-oh-gee). Play lots of rhyming games, can you hear the way these words all sound the same "Trick, Stick, Click" – that's right they all have "ck" or "ick" sounds in them.
- Clap syllables out so they start to understand how words are broken down, dog has one syllable and equals one clap, the word person has two syllables (per-son) and equals two claps. Being able to understand syllables is a precursor for being able to understand how words are structured and written.

Social and Emotional Milestones –

- Rules Police! At this age children really start to become aware of and enforce rules. They can become quite bossy or "tell" on people who are breaking the rules, mostly this comes from trying to make sense of the world and all of the rules and find it hard to manage exceptions. Their thinking is quite concrete and rigid and this is also coupled with increased ability to compare and contrast things and them starting to develop a moral and value system, which makes them quite focussed on "right versus wrong".

- Emotional regulation is improving so they are better able to play cooperative games and also better able to cope with winning and losing.
- Their play has become more complex, and friendships are increasingly prioritized. Children of this age are starting to really feel a sense of belonging and self-esteem associated with having a peer group, this can result in acting like their friends to seek approval (you might see fun new phrases or materialism as they try to fit in – wanting what their friends have). They can also start to show jealousy when others encroach on their friendships.
- Approval! Our five to six-year olds are really seeking approval at this stage of life, from their friends, teachers and parents. They want you to take them and their ideas seriously, and can still be capable of sulking and tantrums when they don't feel heard or acknowledged.

Supporting Social and Emotional Milestones

- Watch tv shows and read books with them and ask them to identify the emotions of different characters. Not only that, ask them why they came to that answer. We want our kids tapping into empathy, which is the ability to understand another person's feelings/perspectives.
- Play games with rules and teach them the art of being a good loser (and winner). Our children need to become resilient and cope with losing, but they also need to win with grace. Either circumstance can be challenging for our little people, because of course they want to win, but at this age there is an added complexity of wanting to retain and protect their friendships and also learn about cooperation for the benefit of a group they align with. So, teaching them how to react in either situation

with dignity is very important. Talk to them about what it feels like to lose, encourage them to learn or pull something from the situation to help them next time or teach them positive phrases to practice

- I lost and that made me feel really sad, but I know that for the next game I need to practice my catching skills.
- I lost and that makes me feel mad, so I'm going to take some deep breaths and sit quietly in my room for a few minutes until I feel like talking.
- It was disappointing that I didn't win, but I'm going to try again next time.

- Encourage dress up and play with different character roles, especially those in helping professions; nurses, doctors, vets, police officers, fire fighters, teachers etc. When they step into these helping roles it helps give them the freedom to play out and explore empathy, compassion and helping.

BUILDING A STRONG RELATIONSHIP WITH YOUR 5-6 YEAR OLD

At this age your child is really seeking approval from you and other key people in their lives. It can be very easy for this need for approval to become entwined with their self-esteem, in particular when we use praise as a reward, or use terms like "good boy" or "good girl" to appreciate their behavior. It's not to say that we can't appreciate them, but we need to be careful in what behaviors we promote, namely in how we give positive attention. When we aren't specific and we say "good girl/boy" we aren't giving any details to our child about the exact behaviors that we appreciate or are socially appropriate (so they don't know what behavior to replicate or what expectations they have achieved), but also, we are only acknowledging the outcome, not the input. For example, if your child is trying to tie their shoes and after multiple attempts, they get it right, and you say *"Great job, good boy/girl"* they learn only you were pleased with the outcome, not their efforts to get it right. You could vary it slightly and have a completely different outcome *"I noticed how hard you tried to tie your shoes, great job!"*

It's also very tempting to heap praise on your child, because you want them to repeat positive behaviors; however, this reward of you saying how wonderful they are and the self-esteem boost they receive in result is what drives their behavior forward. Wanting to please someone or relying on an external person to tell them they have done a good job can be problematic going forward, because they aren't driven within themselves to succeed and rely on others input to feel good about themselves, or they may easily give up if they don't receive the praise they crave. Instead you can offer similar feedback and acknowledgement as above, instead of heaping on the praise and really trying to get your child to take ownership and pride in their own behaviors/choices: *"I can see how hard you tried, and you kept going until you finally built that block tower."* Praise can also be about being interested *"I can see you have been painting, can you tell me about what you were painting and the colors you picked?"* or it could even be getting them to identify what it felt like for them to do a good job *"You won that running race, what did it feel like for you?"*

To instil a sense of pride in your child, and also to get them thinking about you all working together as a family (which improves connection and a strong relationship), it's important to get your child involved in looking after their activities of daily living and also contributing to the running of the family house. I don't mean chores (which come with a reward in return for doing a job around the house), I mean a genuine contribution to the family and home. Children of this age love to be seen as responsible and helpful, so sit down together and figure out what they can do for themselves (I can pick my own clothes, brush my teeth and put my pjs in the wash) as well as looking at ways they can help the entire family (putting their cutlery and bowl/plate in the sink after using, tidying their bedroom, packing up their toys after they play). When children see themselves as capable, they feel good about themselves and confident in their abilities to look after themselves. They also feel a sense of pride in helping out the family and feel more connected to you when they have a role in the family and they know that they are contributing.

THE ART OF TAKING A MINDFUL WALK (ACTIVITY)

Mindfulness is a bit of a buzzword, essentially it is about learning a set of skills that help us bring awareness to the present moment (rather than focusing on our thoughts, worries, or the future). It can help us remain calm, increase our focus and gives us the mental space to make purposeful decisions rather than reacting. You also develop the lifelong skill of being able to quieten your busy mind and better regulate your emotions. This is a skill which benefits adults and children of all ages. With this in mind, I'd like to introduce you to the notion of taking a "Mindful Walk".

So how does one mindfully walk?

Arrange a trip to somewhere quiet (with minimal people around) that has beautiful views/scenery. It could be a local park, river, beach, forest/bushland. This activity can be done with either comfortable walking shoes or bare feet, depending on the terrain and safety of the area. Before you get started, read these steps and make a plan of action, but please know that there is no right or wrong way of doing it. Instead set yourself the goal of paying attention to your thoughts, letting them go and bringing awareness to your body during the activities. This is how we become "present". If you are bringing your child along for a mindful walk, encourage them to focus on the feelings in their body and the steps they are taking...you might even "get them in the zone" by doing a calm breathing activity first.

Find a Calm Place to Take a Mindful Walk

If you are mindfully walking with your child, ask these questions aloud, and give them a minute or two (or less if they have a shorter attention span) to consider your question. If you are walking alone simply reflect and consider the sensations in your body as you follow the mindful walking guide.

1. You want to start by focusing on your feet, so first bring attention to the weight of your feet on the ground and think about the sensation of standing. Is the ground even? Is it hot or cold? Soft or firm?
2. If you have shoes on can you notice the sensation of your socks? Or the pressure of your shoes? If you don't have shoes on then try to wiggle your toes and feel the sensation of the ground beneath you. What does it feel like, is it rough, soft, gritty, hard?
3. The next stage is taking very slow steps (between 10 and 20 depending on your or your child's concentration level). I want you to think about how your feet move when you take a step (pressure moving from the toes, to the ball of the foot and lifting the heel).
4. After 10/20 steps focusing on your feet stepping, I want you to now think about the movement of your knees when you walk. How do they bend and stretch or straighten as you step? Can you feel the muscles in your legs that are used to make the knee bend?
5. After 10/20 steps focusing on your knees I want you to place your hands on your belly (between the belly button and the rib cage). Try to pay attention to the way your belly rises and falls as you breathe. I encourage you to take deep breaths through your nose and breathe out through your mouth. Once you have mastered this

breathing, take 10/20 slow steps and notice the pattern of your breathing. Then adapt this and take 10/20 fast steps and see if you notice any difference to your breathing.

6. You can repeat these patterns as many times as you like (or however long your interest/concentration will last for).

This is only one example which shows how easy it is to incorporate mindfulness activities into your daily life. This activity can also be done in the home, in the garden, and with regular household objects or actions (like pouring a glass of water, or playing with playdough). And whilst the outcome is that you and your child will experience a sense of calm, better emotional regulation and the ability to make purposeful decisions as opposed to rash reactions, this is not the only intention of mindfulness practices.

Enjoy the time you have spent creating a sense of presence. Help your child to carve out space in their daily life that isn't focussed on worries and future planning. You are teaching them that they can enjoy a full life that isn't fulfilling because it's busy and jam-packed, a life that is full simply because they are present in the moment and are attuned to the positives.

FEELINGS IN MY BODY (ACTIVITY)

For a printable resource of this Feelings in My Body chart, head to www.littleones.co/3to6years

The aim of this activity is to get your child connected to what different emotions feel like, and where they notice these feelings in their bodies. Being able to correctly identify emotions gives our children a sense of power and confidence because they understand what is happening to them, but when they can identify their feelings it also gives them a lot of useful information about how to cope, i.e. we deal with anger differently than we do sadness.

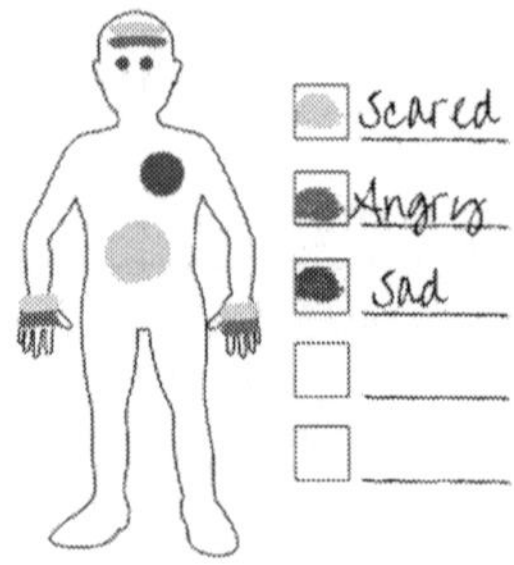

Step 1:

It's important to know that there are no right or wrong answers. Your child can pick any color, or choose anywhere in the body that they notice their emotions. They also don't have to fill in all of the boxes, or additionally they could add more boxes if they wish.

Step 2:

Grab a bunch of different coloured pens, pencils, crayons for your child to use.

Step 3:

Ask your child to think about different feelings, if they need a prompt start with key feelings; happy, sad, angry, scared. Children of different ages will have a better understanding of complex feelings so don't pressure them to accept or identify any particular emotions. Whatever list they come up with is perfect, help them (if they need it) to write down the list of feelings on the lines.

Step 4:

Get your child to color in a box using a color that represents the different emotions that they

identified. Again, there is no right or wrong answer here.

Step 5:

Next, get your child to think about where they feel particular emotions in their body, and using the corresponding color, get them to color in the area on the body. If you need to prompt them you could explore some prompts; being scared could leave us feeling sick (tummy might get colored in), their hands might shake (hands get coloured in), when we are sad we might cry (eyes are colored in) etc. Remember everybody notices their feelings occurring in different places in their bodies so there is no correct answer.

Taking the activity further:

Now your child has a better understanding of their feelings, you can ask them about different coping strategies once they have identified their feeling. You can also ask them questions to help you understand their emotions better too *"Oh I see that when you are angry you feel it in your hands, do they feel hot or are they shaky?"* or *"Do you know what sorts of things make you feel sad?"*. You could also laminate a blank activity form and stick it on the fridge, each day before or after school or at times of stress you could get them in the habit of filling in the body so they can communicate their feelings with you easily.

CHORES BY AGE

Between 3-6 years old, your little one is well capable of participating in household chores. This gives them a real sense of responsibility and makes them feel like a contributing part of the family. Here is a list of appropriate chores by age, which is also available as a downloadable chart at www.littleones.co/3to6years

2-3 Years • Wipe table after meals • Pack away toys and books • Help put dishes away • Help get mail • Help feed pets	**4-5 Years** Previous chores plus: • Set table • Clear table • Empty cutlery from dishwasher • Put own laundry away • Get mail • Feed pets • Dust surfaces
6-8 Years Previous chores plus: • Sweep floor • Pack and unpack	**8-10 Years** Previous chores plus: • Vacuum floor • Wash dishes

dishwasher • Dry dishes • Fold laundry • Pack school lunches • Help cook dinner • Empty trash • Water garden	• Cook a simple dinner • Clean shower • Wash car • Unpack groceries • Hang up washing • Mop floors

WE'D LOVE TO HELP YOU MORE!

Hopefully the comprehensive information and methods in this book have brought some light to the end of the tunnel for you and your family. Parenting is really tough, we know that because we're parents too and are still right in the thick of it ourselves.

There is hope! And we can do it together.

To that end, we have a ton of additional information and articles on our website if you're interested in further reading about a whole range of baby, toddler and child sleep and wellness topics.

And then of course we have our incredible Little Ones App, inside which are detailed programs, schedules, trackers, methods, troubleshooting, advice and live sleep consultants for babies from birth to 3 years old. If you have a baby or toddler at home, or know someone who does, head to our website and enjoy a 10% discount on our App subscription by using the code LITTLEONES4SLEEP.

We'd love to see you at www.littleones.co and continue helping you and your family towards better sleep and more confident parenting.

littleONES
The Baby Sleep Experts

BIBLIOGRAPHY

https://www.kidshealth.org.nz/bedwetting

https://www.mayoclinic.org/diseases-conditions/bed-wetting/symptoms-causes/syc-20366685

Anderson, J. E. (1955). "Review of the construction of reality in the child". Psychological Bulletin. 52 (6): 526–8. doi:10.1037/h0039645.

Bower, T. G. R. (1974). Development in infancy. San Francisco: Freeman.

Dornam, H., & Dornam, C. (2002) The social toddler, Richmond: The Children's Project Ltd, www.childrenproject.co.uk.

Fishel, A. H. (1987) Children's Adjustment in Divorced Families. Youth & Society 19:2, pages 173-196.

King Mize, L., & McMullen, M. (2000) Creative Solutions to Families in Transition. Journal of Family Psychotherapy 10 (4), 21-35.

Lindon, J. (2006) Care and caring matter: young children learning through care, London: Early Education.

Lindon, J. (2009) Parents as partners, London: Practical Pre-School Books

Lindon, J. (2008) What does it mean to be one (two, three, four, five), a set of five books, London: Practical Pre-School Books.

Murray, L., & Andrews, L. (2000) The social baby, Richmond: The Children's Project Ltd.

Piaget, J. (1977). Gruber, Howard E.; Vonèche, J. Jacques. (eds.). The essential Piaget. London: Routledge and K. Paul. ISBN 978-0710087782. OCLC 3813049.

Australian Government Department of Health and Aging (2010). Move and play every day: National physical activity recommendations for children 0-5 years. Canberra: Commonwealth of Australia. Retrieved 12 February 2020 from https://www1.health.gov.au/internet/main/publishing.nsf/Content/F01F92328EDADA5BCA257BF0001E720D/$File/FS%200-5yrs.PDF.

Carter, R.G., & Feigelman, S. (2019). The preschool years. In R. Kliegman & J. St Geme (Eds), Nelson textbook of pediatrics (21st edn, pp. 143-145). Philadelphia, PA: Saunders Elsevier.

Centers for Disease Control and Prevention (2012). Developmental milestones. Atlanta, GA: CDC. Retrieved 12 February 2020 from http://www.cdc.gov/ncbddd/actearly/milestones/.

Conti-Ramsden, G., & Durkin, K. (2012). Language development and assessment in the preschool period. Neuropsychology Review, 22(4), 384-401. doi: 10.1007/s11065-012-9208-z.

Dosman, C.F., Andrews, D., & Goulden, K.J. (2012). Evidence-based milestone ages as a framework for developmental surveillance. Paediatrics and Child Health, 17(10), 561-568. doi: 10.1093/pch/17.10.561.

Gerber, R.J., Wilks, T., & Erdie-Lalena, C. (2011). Developmental milestones 3: Social-emotional development. Pediatrics in Review, 32(12), 533-536. doi: 10.1542/pir.32-12-533.

Gerber, R.J., Wilks, T., & Erdie-Lalena, C. (2010). Developmental milestones: Motor development. Pediatrics in Review, 31(7), 267-277. doi: 10.1542/pir.31-7-267.

Johnson, S. (2012). A clinical handbook on child development paediatrics. Chatswood, NSW: Elsevier Australia.

Lawrence, R., & Bateman, N. (2013). 12 minute consultation: An evidence-based approach to the management of a child with speech and language delay. Clinical Otolaryngology, 38(2), 148-153. doi: 10.1111/coa.12082.

National Scientific Council on the Developing Child (2004). Young children develop in an environment of relationships. Working paper no. 1. Cambridge, MA: Centre on the Developing Child, Harvard University. Retrieved 12 February 2020 from http://developingchild.harvard.edu/wp-content/uploads/2004/04/Young-Children-Develop-in-an-Environment-of-Relationships.pdf.

Oberklaid, F., & Drever, K. (2011). Is my child normal? Milestones and red flags for referral. Australian Family Physician, 40(9), 666-670. Retrieved 12 February 2020 from http://www.racgp.org.au/download/documents/AFP/2011/September/201109oberklaid.pdf.

Oberklaid, F., & Kaminsky, L. (2006). Your child's health. Melbourne: Hardie Grant.

Skolnick Weisburg, K. (2015). Pretend play. WIREs Cognitive Science, 6(3), 249-261. doi: 10.1002/wcs.1341.

Sharma, A., & Cockerill, H. (2014). Mary Sheridan's from birth to five years: Children's developmental progress (4th edn). London: Routledge.

Victorian Department of Education and Early Childhood Development (2011). Child health record.Melbourne: Victorian Government.

Wilks, T., Gerber, R.J., & Erdie-Lalena, C. (2010). Developmental milestones: Cognitive development.Pediatrics in Review, 31(9), 364-367. doi: 10.1542/pir.31-9-364.

PRAISE FOR AUTHOR

I recommend this to any struggling young mother on my path. The book for 3-6 year olds has been one I've been coming back to so often when I run into an issue or don't know how to properly respond (night terrors, bedtime struggles, introducing shared room...). Also the info on development and building strong relationships with your kids has been a great affirmation that my husband and I are on the right track. Recommend to everyone, it's worth every dollar.

- FEMKE

Little Ones saved my sanity!
I am obsessed with the Little Ones app! I have now turned into that nutty person who raves on about it and advises everyone with a baby to get it. My favorite part about Little Ones is that I can get help anytime day or night. Being able to get instant advice, troubleshooting and support on contingency plans when our routine goes awry is incredible. In only a few short weeks, my 4 month old has gone from only sleeping in 30 minute bursts during the day and he is now sleeping 12.5 hours overnight and is the most settled and happy he has ever been. I feel like I have my sanity back and I can be the calm, supportive mother that I want to be for my baby.

- RACHAEL, AUSTRALIA

So thankful for this app!!
I got this app for my second baby who struggled with sleep a lot more than my first. I had already trained her to self soothe but she STILL wasn't napping longer than 35 minutes! I couldn't figure it out and felt like I was going crazy! She was always screaming and tired. The very first day I tried this schedule, she napped for 2 HOURS at the lunch nap! I couldn't believe it!! I love using the tracker on the app - it is such a useful tool! All the troubleshooting tips are extremely helpful when things don't go as planned. I love that I am now about to get out and about with my baby and toddler in the morning, knowing they'll both have naps at the same time right after lunch. I really appreciate being able to use the program just for how long I need it. Thank you so much!

- ANNALISE, USA

Little Ones app was a Godsend for me! I am a new mommy and was going off of advice from everyone around me. Following my baby girl's cues for feeds/naps unfortunately did not work and every day was a challenge because every day was different. I love that there is now a routine in which we know what's coming next. More importantly, my baby girl is always super HAPPY and everyone notes how calm she is. This app helps both babies and mommies get good rest and enjoy the magical journey. Just knowing one can get quick answers from sleep experts is also such a relief. I will be and have been recommending this to all the expecting mommies. Thank you Little Ones!

- ANUDEEP

Printed in Great Britain
by Amazon

12732532R00077